THE KNEE

PROBLEMS AND PREVENTION
A Self-help Guide

Vivian Grisogono

JOHN MURRAY
Albemarle Street, London

© Vivian Grisogono 1998

First published in 1998
by John Murray (Publishers) Ltd.,
50 Albemarle Street, London W1X 4BD

617 582
Gris

A catalogue record for this book is available from the British Library

Readers are advised to seek professional help in any case of injury. The author and publishers cannot be held responsible for readers' injuries in any circumstances.

ISBN 0-7195-5538 8

Typeset in 10 on 12.5pt Sabon

Printed and bound in Great Britain by Butler and Tanner Limited, Frome

Contents

Acknowledgements

Very many friends have helped by lending their knees, talents and expertise, and I am very grateful to them, especially Kate Andrew, Michael Bartlett, Nigel Cullen, George Dowd, Peter Gardiner, Richard Gardner, Basil Helal, John Ireland, Gareth Jones, Charles King, Sue Murray, Ross Norman, Shola Roper, Colin Roshier and Marla Williams.

As ever, I have to thank everyone at John Murray for their continuing kindness, friendship and support, and most notably Gail Pirkis, whose ability to cajole, bully and persuade in the nicest way possible makes her a specially efficacious editor.

Who gets knee problems?

1

Anyone of any age and either sex can suffer injury, pain, inflammation, infection or disease affecting one or both knees. Writing about the knee over twelve years ago, I calculated that I had treated over 1,200 knee problems in eight years. Now, after more than twenty years in practice as a chartered physiotherapist I have long since given up counting. Knee problems are still the most common injury among sports players, and high on the problem list among non-sporting patients.

This book aims to help you understand how the knee works and why it can go wrong, so that you can learn how to deal with knee problems properly, or, better still, prevent them. It is a self-help book which gives suggestions as to what you should do in different situations when your knees hurt, which type of practitioner you might consult or be referred to, the questions you should ask, and which treatments might be offered. You will also be able to use the suggestions for protective and remedial exercises safely, provided you follow the guidelines to the letter.

This is not a manual for self-diagnosis or self-treatment. Trying to guess at the diagnosis of your problem will only cause you

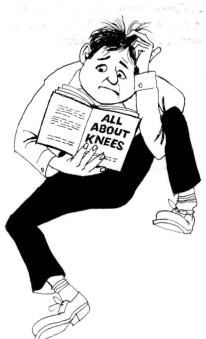

Self-diagnosis only leads to confusion

trouble. Diagnosis, assessment and treatment are specialized and must always be left to appropriate qualified practitioners.

As the book is written primarily for lay people, it is not referenced in the way a technical text would be. However, for those readers interested in reading in more detail about the scientific and clinical background to what I have written, selected books and articles are listed under topic headings at the end of the book.

CASE STUDIES FOR HOPE

In almost every case of knee pain, it is possible to improve matters, so long as the cause of the problem is identified and an accurate treatment strategy applied and followed. This applies equally to children, top sports players, fit and unfit middle-aged people and pensioners, male and female.

Accurate rehabilitation is the key to recovery. Any number of examples can be found among my patients: the 24-year-old accountant, a competitive cyclist, who suffered chronic problems in his right knee and had several operations over two years, but was able to cycle again; the 36-year-old businessman who had suffered knee pain for twenty years, having been a competitive skier, who was cured after three months; the 46-year-old lady who, having injured her right knee skiing, had an operation to repair her torn cruciate ligament, and was able to dance and ski again; the 77-year-old lady, a survivor from Dachau concentration camp, with a long history of arthritis in her knees and frequent falls, who recovered to be able to walk up and down stairs and dig her garden without pain.

Even after seemingly catastrophic injuries, it is possible to make a full, long-term recovery, as the following case studies illustrate.

Successful return to top squash

Ross Norman was a successful professional squash player, ranked number seven in the world, when he injured his left knee at the age of 24. He made a slightly awkward landing on concrete from a parachute jump, and felt the inner side of his knee give. Swelling quickly appeared all round the joint, and there was bruising down the inner side.

Initially, the local casualty department put the leg in plaster, but after a couple of weeks Ross came under the care of a sports specialist orthopaedic surgeon, who repaired his posterior cruciate ligament, which had totally ruptured. The surgeon gave him a fifty-fifty chance of ever playing squash again.

After the operation, Ross was kept in bed in hospital for six weeks, with the knee bent and the shin-bone held forward in traction by a pin. He was then allowed up with a brace to protect the knee. Two months after surgery, Ross attended for an out-patient physiotherapy session. He was now allowed to try to straighten his knee, but had to wait for another week before trying to bend it beyond a right angle. The session consisted of manual therapy to help the knee's extension movement, manipulations to free the kneecap, mobilizing exercises using free-wheeling on a high saddle on an exercise bicycle, and a basic remedial exercise programme, including specific work for the hamstring muscles, to do at home.

The following week I accompanied Ross to his sports club to set out a progressive remedial exercise and physical training schedule using the equipment in the gymnasium. He was able to start aerobic training using swimming and the static bicycle. He worked out in the gymnasium for about two and a half hours every day. When he attended for physiotherapy nine days later, he was still about 15 degrees short of being able to straighten his knee, but bending had improved to about 100 degrees. The early physiotherapy sessions consisted of mobility work for flexion on the exercise bicycle with the saddle lowered, passive stretching to bend the knee in the stomach-lying position, and electrical muscle stimulation using a faradic stimulator for the vastus medialis obliquus in the sitting position with the knee supported over a pillow. Balancing

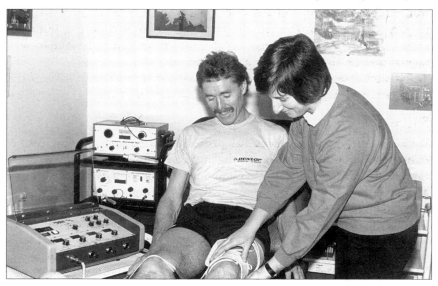

The author treating squash player Ross Norman with electrical neuromuscular stimulation for the vastus medialis obliquus

exercises started with simply standing on the left leg, then standing and bending and straightening the knee slightly, progressing to doing the same things standing on the wobble board.

The post-operative rehabilitation period lasted three months, during which Ross received eight treatment sessions. Each session consisted of treatments to help the functional improvement, and further instructions and goal-setting for the self-help programme which was the key to recovery.

About six weeks after starting his rehabilitation programme, Ross began to run for ten minutes or so every second day, and he started doing solo practices on the squash court, hitting straight up and down the wall. He gradually increased his running to about twenty minutes and was doing more complex movements like running backwards and sprinting exercises on the squash court. I discouraged him from road-running every day, added half-squats on the left leg to the remedial programme, and recommended more varied practice on the squash court, plus leg-lunging movements in front of a mirror to improve his co-ordination.

Four months after the operation, Ross was able to play squash competitively again, which was an urgent need as it was his sole source of income. Three years after his accident, Ross became world squash champion. He continued to play top-level squash for nearly ten more years, was still ranked in the world's top ten at the age of 36, and was ranked twelve when he retired from the professional game.

Ross's left knee suffered only one setback, when he had to run to catch a boat wearing loose flip-flop sandals, some six years after the original accident. The surgeon injected the painful gastrocnemius tendon at the back of the knee, and Ross had three physiotherapy treatment sessions consisting of massage, diadynamic therapy, ice, ultrasound and electrical muscle stimulation for the vastus medialis obliquus. The problem was resolved completely within ten days.

Ross continued to enjoy a wide range of sporting activities, including water-skiing and para-gliding. Despite minor injuries elsewhere, the left knee remained stable, allowing Ross to continue competitive representative squash even after retiring from the professional circuit.

Fourteen years after his accident, Ross said that he had only hoped for five years of professional squash when he re-started playing after the operation. He paid full tribute to the skill of the orthopaedic surgeon who rescued his knee, as without accurate surgery he would certainly not have been able to play again.

Beyond the surgery, Ross's success was due most of all to his motivation and the disciplined way in which he followed through his rehabilitation programme. He has continued to do remedial knee exercises consistently within his training schedule, and this has certainly been a crucial factor in preventing any deterioration in the joint or secondary problems.

Trauma recovery and the show went on

A 22-year-old actress tripped and fell on to her right knee on concrete, and felt immediate acute pain over the bony tibial tubercle just below the knee. There was no noticeable swelling at the time, but the knee was enlarged by the next day, when she came to me for physiotherapy treatment. The tibial tubercle was exquisitely painful to touch, and the vastus medialis obliquus muscle was inhibited.

I had treated this patient two years previously, when she had had an operation on the same knee to clear the back of the kneecap, and she had been pain-free in the intervening period.

For this new injury, I treated her with very gentle massage and electrical muscle stimulation for the vastus medialis obliquus. I asked the patient to resume her remedial exercise programme, concentrating on co-ordination for the vastus medialis obliquus muscle and gentle stretching movements for the front-thigh muscles. She was also advised to use arnica or a heparinoid cream over the tender area, and to wear knee pads when rehearsing for her next show, in which she had to fall on to her knees. Following the treatment session, the patient recovered very quickly using the self-help programme, and was able to perform in the show without any problems.

Long-term injury recovery

A 58-year-old health professional had suffered from right knee pain for some years. There had been several episodes of trauma: a bad fall while the patient was still at school, another fall while skiing when she was in her twenties, and a direct knock in a car accident when she was about 50. The knee had always been slightly painful, but the pain had become much worse following a fall some seven months before she came to me for physiotherapy treatment. She had been receiving chiropractic treatment for three or four years. Her job was very sedentary, and she enjoyed walking and playing recreational tennis, but was increasingly hampered by pain and stiffness after any kind of exercise.

When I first saw this patient, her right knee was visibly swollen, it clicked a lot, and she could not bend it fully to crouch down. I treated her with massage to the back of the knee, which was very tight, electrical muscle stimulation for the vastus medialis obliquus, and stretching techniques for the front-thigh muscles. I set her an overall programme of self-help care, and requested that she should be referred to a specialist orthopaedic surgeon by her general practitioner.

Within three weeks, the surgeon performed an arthroscopy and removed a torn part of the medial semilunar cartilage. At operation, it was noted that there was degenerative damage over the inner part of the knuckle (condyle) of the thigh-bone. When I saw the patient six days after the operation she was already back at work, but was experiencing pain over the inner side of the knee, and the joint felt as restricted as before. I treated her once a week, using massage and manual therapy to ease the knee and help regain the movement, and electrical muscle stimulation for the vastus medialis obliquus muscle (see p.147). The patient followed the remedial exercise programme for stability and mobility (see p.155), took care of her circulation (see p.177), and tried to avoid any irritant foods (see p.46). To help the knee to bend, she used an exercise bicycle without loading and gradually lowered the saddle (see p.155).

After eight weeks, one of the stitches had failed to dissolve and became infected, the knee was slightly inflamed, and the patient was given antibiotics by her GP. A few days after finishing the antibiotics, her knee was feeling better again and the patient went out for the evening, ate a very rich meal with champagne and wine, and danced. As a result, the joint became very hot, reddened and acutely painful. It took three weeks for the knee to recover from this setback, which had a bad effect on the patient's confidence, but after that progress was steady.

Treatment sessions were reduced to one every three weeks, as the mobility and strength of the knee gradually improved and the patient was able to walk further and do more. Four months after the operation, she played her first game of tennis, although another month was needed before she had the confidence to run on court. She was still very wary of crouching down, although she could bend the knee quite well by this time. She then had a car accident, and hurt her left knee, but this recovered quickly following one physiotherapy session. The patient was encouraged to think positively and to maintain her remedial exercises and self-care measures, and she was soon able to resume all her normal activities.

Two years later, she was still able to work, play tennis and go walking with only slight reminders of her right knee problem, which was an excellent result in view of the long-standing damage in the joint.

Promising young tennis player

Shola Roper was 15 and growing fast when his right knee suddenly gave way. He was high jumping, and the tibial tubercle just below his knee broke off in an avulsion fracture. He fell down and could not get up, although he felt surprisingly little pain.

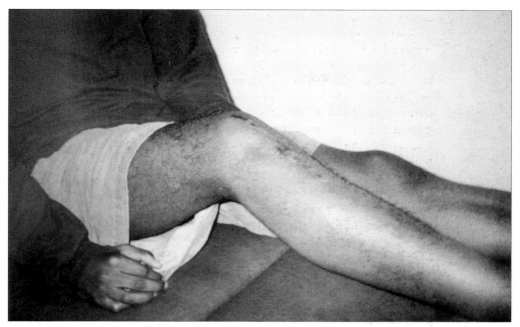

Shola Roper's knee movements were severely restricted

Over three years earlier, he had suffered knee pain in the patellar tendon and tibial tubercle, first on the left side, then on the right. He had grown significantly over six months, and had been playing a lot of tennis on hard cement courts wearing trainers. Initially he noticed pain after playing, but then the knee became painful on walking, especially up stairs, so he came to me for a physiotherapy session. Shola was very tall and slim, and his leg muscles were noticeably weak and inflexible. He found it difficult to stand on his right leg and go up and down on his toes, and when his front-thigh muscles were stretched as he lay on his stomach his heels were about five inches away from his bottom. His hip mobility was fairly good, without any signs of irritation, but squatting down hurt the right knee, and the right vastus medialis obliquus was weakened.

I gave Shola a self-help rehabilitation programme for Osgood-Schlatter's condition: this consisted of ice applications for the tibial tubercle region, remedial exercises to improve flexibility and strength in all the leg muscle groups, rest from painful sports such as tennis and football, and continuing painless activities. A report was written for his school teachers detailing what he should and should not do. Shola was also encouraged to use different sports shoes for different playing surfaces, by investing in cheaper, simpler types of sports shoes and

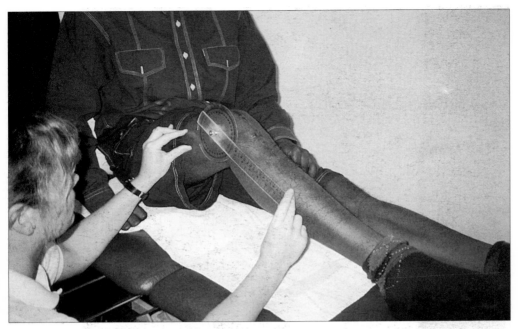

Goniometer measurements were used for motivation

reinforcing them with protective insoles.

The problem settled within about four months without further intervention, and Shola was able to return to full sporting activities without setbacks. A few days before the avulsion fracture of his right tibial tubercle he had noticed some pain over the bone after playing tennis and football, but not enough to worry him. When the tibial tubercle broke, Shola was taken to hospital and the bone was fixed back surgically with a staple. He then started rehabilitation treatment at the hospital, doing standard remedial exercises including straight-leg-raises, but he made little headway. Six months after the operation, Shola came to me for treatment. He was walking stiff-legged, and had been unable to attend school for the whole period because of his disability. Extension was fair, although he was unable to straighten the knee fully, but bending was severely limited – to only 38 degrees sitting up, 18 degrees actively and 28 degrees passively when he lay on his stomach. He naturally feared that his knee would 'burst' again if he forced it to move, and that it would never get better.

Shola attended for physiotherapy treatment three or four times a week for six months. The treatment plan was to encourage Shola to regain maximum knee function by restoring his confidence, while monitoring

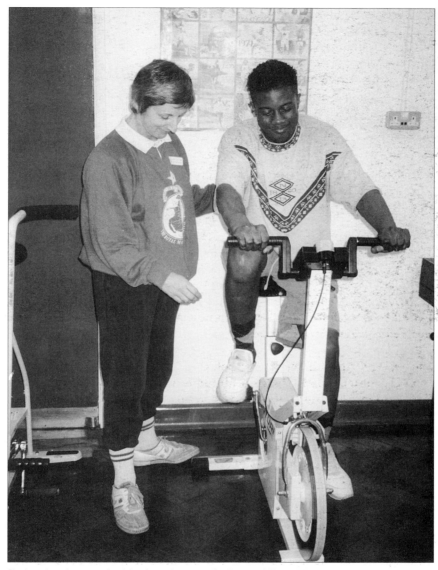

Shola using the exercise bicycle to increase flexion mobility, with encouragement from the author

him carefully just in case further surgical intervention was needed. The programme consisted of manual therapy to mobilize the kneecap and normalize the sensation of the patellar tendon; massage for the extended, tight scar; electrical muscle stimulation for the vastus medialis obliquus;

assisted movements, mobilizing techniques and proprioceptive neuromuscular facilitation to improve knee mobility and efficiency; exercises using gymnasium equipment; and stretching and stabilizing exercises which were also to be done daily at home.

Measurements and verbal encouragement were used to provide motivation and reassurance. Apart from measuring the range of flexion with a goniometer at regular intervals, the saddle height for free-wheeling bending was recorded at each session. Shola used the seated leg press machine not only for strengthening the thigh muscles concentrically and eccentrically, but also to increase the range of right knee flexion by gradually letting the weights release further as he bent the knees on the reverse movement. It took about eight weeks for the right knee to bend sufficiently to control the weights back to the starting position, after which he was able to do the leg press exercise with the right leg on its own.

From the start Shola used the mini-trampoline for balance and co-ordination exercises, to regain the feeling of normal walking and eventually running. He used the step machine, rowing ergometer, hip abduction and adduction machine and upper body weights machines for symmetrical exercise and cardiorespiratory fitness, all of which helped him to believe that he could recover. After about six weeks on the

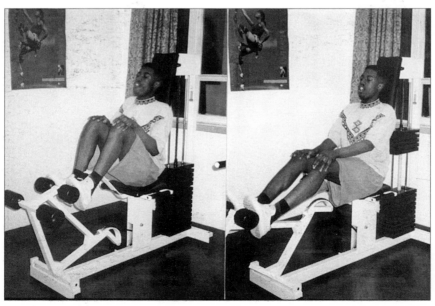

Using the leg press machine for strength and mobility training

programme, Shola was able to start playing tennis on the practice wall. He quickly progressed to practising on court, and was able to start running forwards and sideways in his gym sessions.

After four months, Shola was confident enough to play tennis and basketball. Complex demanding exercises like burpees, squat jumps and lunges were added to the programme. The knee was still slightly stiff, so the treatments to promote flexibility were continued. There were no setbacks during the rehabilitation period, except for a few days when the knee became warm and stiffer after Shola ate some chocolate. After six months, Shola was discharged, as he was fully fit for sports.

He was given maximum reassurance when he was due to have the staple removed from his knee, which was done some ten weeks later. Immediately after the operation, he was very afraid to put his weight through the leg, but after four treatment sessions over one month, consisting of electrical muscle stimulation for vastus medialis obliquus, massage for the scar and manual therapy techniques for mobility, and a few sessions in the rehabilitation gymnasium, he was able to play tennis again without inhibition.

Three years later, the knee had not troubled him at all, and Shola was

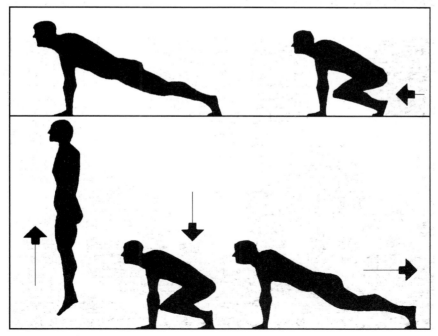

The sequence for burpee jumps (left to right)

playing tennis very successfully alongside his college studies, having won the Middlesex County Under-21 championship and gained the sponsorship which would allow him to pursue his competitive career.

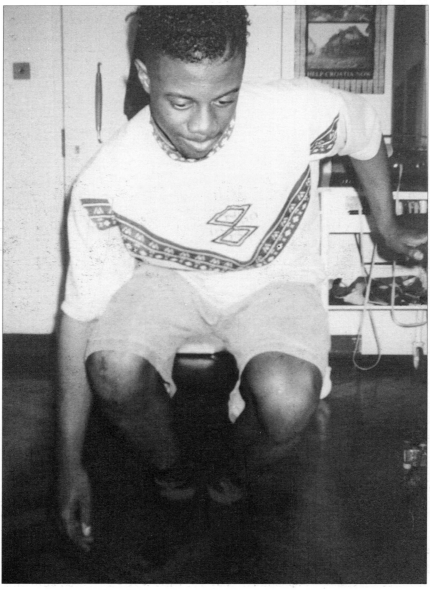

Squatting was a test of confidence and proof of recovery

Common forms of knee abuse

2

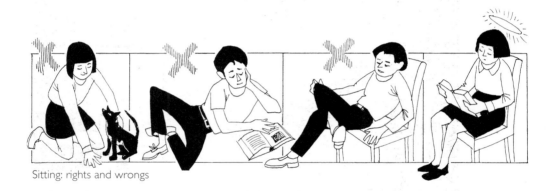

Sitting: rights and wrongs

Θhe knee is constituted to withstand all kinds of pressures and to perform a variety of movements in co-ordination with the rest of the leg. However, it is surprisingly easy to abuse it, through ignorance, misuse or neglect, even in situations which do not seem to carry any obvious risk of harm. Understanding what the risks are is essential to preventing the avoidable knee problems.

POSTURE

Poor postural habits are often established in childhood or the teenage years, so it is especially important for parents, teachers and other responsible adults to make sure that children are encouraged and persuaded to sit and stand as correctly as possible. Bad posture can be acquired by example, as children may copy the way a favoured adult sits or stands. In most cases, distorted postural habits are repeated in the same pattern all the time, so that they feel comfortable and 'normal'. It becomes ever harder to correct the bad habits, because it is difficult to remember to do so, and motivation is lessened by the feeling that correct posture is not pleasant.

Bad posture at any age can be due to poor muscle tone and lack of fitness. It creates asymmetry, causing muscle imbalance and joint distortion. In the growing child this can result in distorted growth patterns, with limitation of normal movement in the affected joints. In the adult, in the worst of cases, there can be pain directly related to joint limitation, and permanent visible deformity.

Sitting

Sitting still for long periods does not do the knees any favours. The flow of blood and synovial fluid is slowed down when you are inactive. Reduction of the circulatory flow also impedes the normal activity of the nerve systems, making the joints and their muscles inefficient. The muscles round the knees are at a disadvantage: the hamstrings are shortened and the key part of the quadriceps group, the vastus medialis muscle, is undermined. Sitting with your legs crossed is even worse, because it distorts the joints asymmetrically.

People of all ages may have the habit of tucking their feet round their chair legs, especially if they are sitting at a desk. This twists the knees, creating strain especially over the medial ligaments on the inner sides of the knees. Many children and some adults like sitting on the floor in the 'frog position', kneeling with their bottom between their heels and their feet splayed sideways. This not only creates rotational distortion at the knees, but seriously compromises the circulation. Sitting with one or both knees twisted and tucked under you is also asking for trouble, as the knees are distorted and their ligaments stressed and compressed. Not only does this create a damaging imbalance in the knees, but it puts the hips and lower back at risk as well.

If you have to sit for long periods, sit straight and symmetrically. Never sit with your legs crossed, either at the knees or at the ankles. Use a cushioned upright chair at the right height for your table or desk. Try to keep your legs moving, and stand up and walk around whenever you can.

Standing

You should avoid standing with one knee slightly bent, as this causes shortening in the tendons behind the knee, especially the hamstrings, and bends the hip on that side, so that it does not bear weight correctly. A persistent tendency to keep one knee bent while standing can result in the knee remaining permanently bent and unable to straighten out fully, with a similar loss of range of movement in the hip. The hip and knee on the other side are overloaded through supporting more than their fair share of your bodyweight. In the long term, there can be wear and tear in either hip or knee because of the unbalanced posture.

Kneeling

When you kneel down the weight of your thighs, trunk, arms and head bears down on to the fronts of your knees. The circulatory flow through your legs is slowed down, partly because your knees are held still in a fixed position, and partly because you are not stimulating the blood flow through normal pressure from the sole of your foot. If you kneel on a hard surface, the compressive effects are much greater than on a soft cushioned surface. The front of the knee is quite bony, but it has some soft fat pads and bursae (natural fluid-filled cysts) which can be irritated by direct pressure.

DRIVING

Driving can create problems if your position is incorrect, or if you keep your legs still in one position for long periods. When you drive, your legs should not be too bent, and certainly not cramped up against the dashboard and steering wheel. If you are very tall, you should avoid vehicles in which the seats do not adjust enough for you to be able to stretch your legs out comfortably. In an automatic car, you should make sure you bend and straighten your left leg at intervals. On long journeys, stop as frequently as possible to get out and stretch your legs by walking around. If your car seat slopes backwards and holds your knees bent, try putting cushions or folded towels on the seat to level it and allow your knees to straighten. When you are a passenger, adjust the seat if possible to allow your legs to straighten out, and move your legs around as much as you can.

If your job involves driving, make sure your vehicle is comfortable. Commercial vehicles such as trucks, vans and taxi-cabs are often designed without much room for adjustment, so if you find you are experiencing problems because the vehicle is not right for you, you should modify the seat as much as you can, or request a change of vehicle.

Diet

You may be surprised to learn that your diet can affect your knees. Foods and drinks which irritate the system can be a direct cause of pain in the knee (see p.46). An inadequate diet, and especially insufficient fluid intake, can contribute to problems in the bones of the knee and the muscles surrounding it.

Shoes

Your shoes can affect the mechanics of your feet, ankles, knees and hips, and alter your body's relationship to gravity.

If you wear very high heels, your bodyweight is tipped forwards and the body's centre of gravity falls further forwards than normal, forcing your knees to bend. In flimsy shoes without a proper heel or shoes with a 'negative heel' which is lower than the forefoot, you are tipped backwards, stretching the muscles on the backs of your legs and making your knees hyperextend.

If the soles of your shoes are hard and rigid, the normal mobility of your feet is blocked, so extra movement is required in the related joints to compensate. As the ankles are stable joints, the extra mobility needed often happens mainly in the knees, placing shearing stresses on the joints. If the related joints cannot compensate properly, you may walk and run with all the leg joints operating stiffly and therefore suffering abnormal loading. This can be a particular problem when walking or running in stiff boots on rough terrain.

Sports shoes should be appropriate to the activity and the surface on which it is played. You need adequate but not excessive grip on smooth surfaces, such as wood, grass, cinders, shale and clay, especially for sports

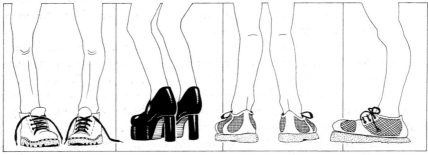

Shoes can hurt knees

which involve sudden changes of direction, such as tennis, badminton and squash. Studs are used for greater security in cross-country running, track events or field games. Smoother-soled shoes may be needed on artificial surfaces which provide a lot of grip, to prevent jarring on the knees. Tennis players, for instance, need several pairs if they play on different court surfaces, such as carpet, grass, cement, clay or the various synthetics. For shock absorption, it is best to use a cushioning insole. The thicker the sole of a sports shoe, the more it impedes normal foot movement and proprioception, which is especially disadvantageous in court games like basketball, netball, badminton, squash and tennis.

INAPPROPRIATE PHYSICAL ACTIVITIES

Inactivity is bad for knees, as for the rest of the human body. The maxim 'If you don't use it, you lose it' applies particularly to the knee's controlling and stabilizing muscles. Too little movement for the knees can lead to painful degenerative arthritis. Sports and physical exercises are generally good for you, but they can be harmful if done wrongly, too often, at the wrong time or in the wrong environment.

Children have to be protected from over-playing, especially during the vulnerable teenage years of growth spurts and bone development. Very young children up to the age of about 11 can undertake a surprising amount of physical activity without ill-effects, even running marathons in creditable times, but their exercise capacity is reduced during growth periods, and they are very likely to suffer overuse injuries if they continue intensive sports. The knee region is especially vulnerable during the early teens.

Children's sporting activities should be balanced, so that children engage in a variety of physical movements, rather than concentrating on only one competitive sport, especially such demanding ones as American football, soccer, swimming or tennis. Active play is better than organized sport, so that the child does not feel forced to participate if he or she does not feel up to it at any given moment.

Sports often create body imbalance which can disrupt the knees. Running, for instance, tends to tighten the hamstrings and hip flexors, drawing the hips and knees into the bent position. The crouching position of squash holds the knees bent under load. Fencing stresses the forward knee and creates imbalance through the whole body. Hurdling jars the lead leg, and stresses the hip and knee of the trail leg rotationally.

Lack of proper preparation can harm the knees. When cold, the knees may be stiff and lack lubrication. A warm-up is essential for the adult

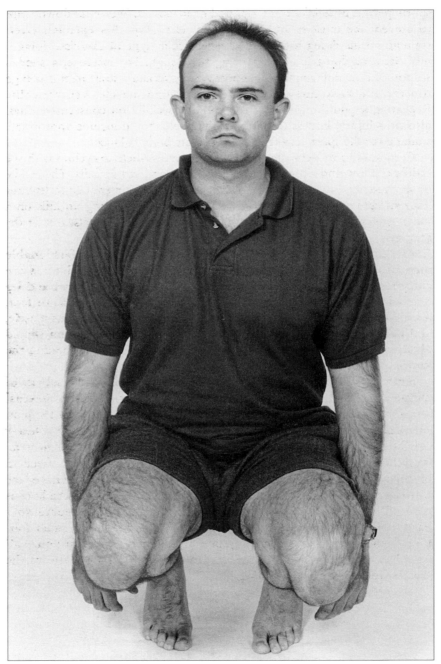

Weightbearing knee-bending is a vital movement for healthy knees

sports player, especially after a period of inactivity. Warming down helps to prevent the muscles and joints from seizing up after exercise. Over-training means doing too much of a particular type of exercise, doing it too often, or doing it without being fit enough. For instance, a sudden session of downhill running is almost certain to cause knee pain if you go too far and have not trained the front-thigh muscles eccentrically. Repeating a punishing session too soon, especially on consecutive days, also risks injury. Fitness training for the adult should include appropriate training for the sport, and exercises to create body balance.

Certain knee movements can cause problems, such as cycling with the saddle too low and sitting down when pedalling hard up hills. The saddle on any moving or static exercise bicycle should be high enough to let your knee straighten out on the downward stroke. When going up hills on a moving bicycle you should always be standing in the pedals, out of the saddle.

Avoiding locking the knees into full extension was a fashionable misconception among fitness instructors for a time. Clients were encouraged not to straighten their knees when using leg press and leg extension machines, or doing aerobics and exercise classes. In fact, avoiding locking out undermines the key vastus medialis obliquus muscle, and can lead directly to kneecap pain syndrome. Full extension should always be the conclusion of any exercise which involves bending the knees.

Squatting down, bending the knees fully has also been the subject of misplaced fear. It threatens knee health only if the knee has an internal injury in which the damaged tissue is irritated or compressed by the joint surfaces as you squat, or through overbalancing while lifting a heavy weight from the deep-squat position. Otherwise, squatting down is an important movement for the knees: it maintains the full degree of freedom of movement, and the cyclical loading lubricates the entire surface of the cartilages. If you cannot squat, the weightbearing area inside the knee is reduced, and you are also unable to use your knees to safeguard your back when lifting objects or weights from the floor. If you squat flat-footed your knee movement may be limited by tightness in your calf muscles, whereas squatting while standing on your toes allows the greatest freedom of knee-bending.

PROTECTIVE SUPPORTS

People who kneel for their work or leisure, such as carpet-layers or gardeners, can suffer knee strains or frictional problems unless they use kneeling pads or cushions.

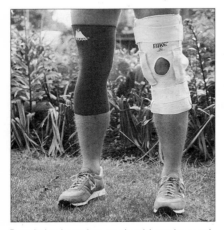

Restrictive knee braces should not be used in order to do activities which would otherwise hurt

Protective clothing or supports should always be used by children or adults taking part in sports or activities which carry a strong risk of physical trauma, such as American football, skateboarding, in-line skating and ice hockey. Supports to protect the knees from knocks should be long enough to enclose the joint completely without cutting into the joint line, and they should be softly padded so that they do not compress the joint or interfere with its freedom of movement.

Knee bandages which enclose the joint should only be used when necessary, usually if the knee is swollen through injury. They are not suitable for injury prevention and should not be used for long periods at a time, as they can have a weakening effect. Weightlifters and powerlifters often bandage their knees tightly when doing deep squats with heavy weights, although it is not clear whether this is protective other than psychologically.

In principle, supports or taping should not be used in order to do activities which would otherwise be too painful. If a knee is potentially unstable after recovering from a major injury, a specially constructed stabilizing brace may be used to protect it in situations of special risk, such as skiing.

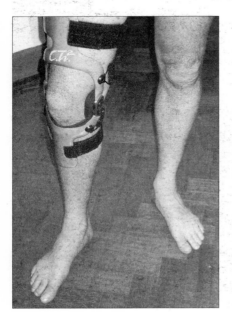

A made-to-measure knee brace offers protection without restriction of movement

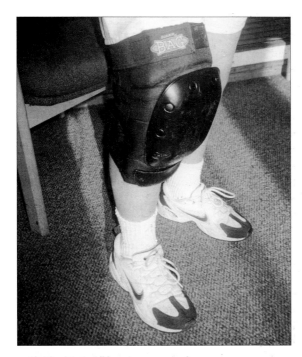

For sports such as
in-line skating, heavy-duty
knee protectors are vital for
cushioning against falls

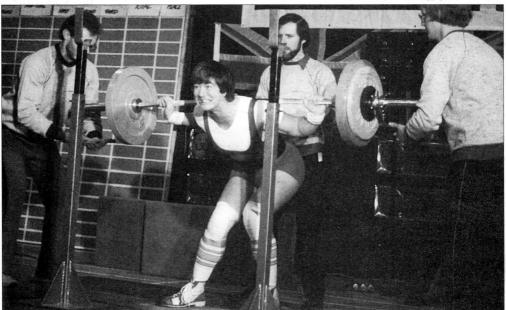

Bandaging or taping the knees for heavy lifting may or may not prevent injury

MIS-TREATED OR UNTREATED INJURIES

Injuries or pains should never be ignored in the adult or the child. Children's knee problems do not necessarily cure themselves, even though they may seem to recover quickly. Injuries, in child or adult, cause muscle inhibition, circulatory disturbance, movement limitation and muscle imbalance. Compensation and secondary overload inevitably happen if full function is not recovered.

Problems have to be treated properly. Rest may ease the immediate symptoms, but will not bring about functional recovery. Trying to get back to demanding sports too soon after an injury is likely to lead to re-injury or secondary problems. The myth that top sportsmen like baseball and soccer players get back more quickly than ordinary people is a bad example. Incomplete recovery from injury is always costly in the short or long term. Rehabilitation under the guidance of a professional practitioner is vital.

How the knee works

3

STRUCTURE OF THE KNEE AND THE KNEECAP JOINTS

The knee is classified as a compound joint, because it consists of two interlinked joints, the tibiofemoral joint between the thigh-bone (femur) and shin-bone (tibia), and the patellofemoral joint between the kneecap and thigh-bone. Technically, the tibiofemoral joint is termed a double condylar joint, while the patellofemoral joint is sellar, because the kneecap is shaped like a saddle that sits across the knuckle of the thigh-bone.

Immediately below the knee is the tibiofibular joint, a tightly bound joint connecting the outer leg-bone with the shin-bone. This is separate from the knee joint itself, but has a functional link with it because the outer (lateral) ligament of the knee and the outer hamstring muscle (biceps femoris) are attached to the head or top of the fibula.

Many people think of the knee as a hinge joint, because its primary actions are to bend (flex) and straighten (extend), but in fact it also has the ability to rotate slightly, a movement which you can perform actively when the knee is bent to a right angle and you turn your foot from side to side, pivoting on your heel. A slight twisting movement happens automatically when the knee moves: your lower leg is turned slightly inwards as you bend the knee, and slightly outwards as you straighten it.

The tibiofemoral joint is load-bearing, and it supports your bodyweight when you are standing up or moving around on your feet. The knee may absorb about three times your bodyweight at every step when you walk, and the jarring pressures are very much greater when you run, jump and hop. Because it is a major weightbearing joint, the knee joint is constructed for stability. However, its structure also allows for a fair degree of freedom of movement, by contrast with the more

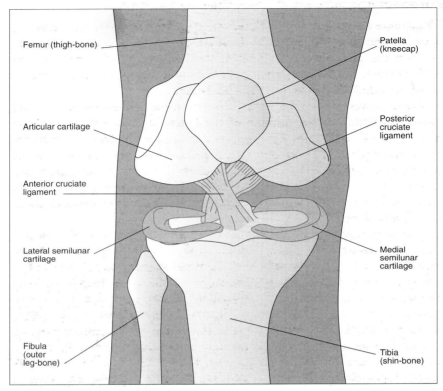

Femur (thigh-bone)

Patella (kneecap)

Articular cartilage

Posterior cruciate ligament

Anterior cruciate ligament

Lateral semilunar cartilage

Medial semilunar cartilage

Fibula (outer leg-bone)

Tibia (shin-bone)

Structures in the right knee seen from the front

rigidly restricted actions of the ankle, for instance. This is why we can do complicated bending and twisting movements using the knees, such as breast-stroke swimming, dancing the Charleston, kicking a football at an angle and moving about in the crouching position.

The kneecap joint does not support the bodyweight directly, and it functions primarily in conjunction with the main knee joint, although it does have a small degree of independent movement. The kneecap is a free-floating bone in the lower end of the quadriceps muscles, and it normally lies over the front of the thigh-bone condyles. The tip of the kneecap lies just above the line of the main knee joint when you are standing up with your legs relaxed. By contracting the thigh muscles very gently, you can draw the kneecap upwards without moving the main knee joint. As the main knee joint straightens, the kneecap automatically glides up over the front of the thigh-bone, and downwards as the knee bends.

Knee configurations and co-ordination patterns

The shape of your knees is determined by several factors, including heredity, the way you have used (or abused) your knees at different stages of your life, any injuries or diseases which have affected your legs, and your posture. The way the knee is shaped has a bearing on its patterns of movement, and therefore on mechanical injuries.

When movements of the leg are described, the convention is to depict them in relation to the midline of the body. Straight-line movements sideways towards or across the midline are termed adduction, movements in the same plane away from the midline abduction. Forward movements are flexion, backward movements extension. Twisting movements are described as internal or medial rotation if the movement is inwards towards the midline, external or lateral rotation when it is outwards away from the midline.

The alignment of the leg bones is subject to variations. In the normal knee, the thigh-bone is placed just about vertically in line over the shin-bone when seen from the side, and slightly diagonally in relation to the shin-bone seen from the front. The angle at which the thigh-bone joins the shin-bone is known as the 'Q-angle'. It is measured where a line drawn from the anterior superior iliac spine at the front of the pelvis down the middle of the thigh-bone to the centre of the kneecap meets a second line through the patellar tendon and tibial tubercle to the middle of the kneecap. Its normal range is considered to be 10–15 degrees. A bigger Q-angle can be due to widely set hips, knock-knee, an outward twist (torsion) of the shin-bone which sets the tibial tubercle further out than normal, or a combination of these factors. A small Q-angle may reflect a narrow pelvis with the hip placed more vertically over the knee, an inward twist on the shin-bone, or bow leg.

The position of the kneecap relative to the tibial tubercle at the top of the shin-bone can be determined by measuring an angle known as the 'A-angle'. This is the intersection of a line drawn vertically downwards through the centre of the kneecap with a second line drawn upwards from the tibial tubercle through the lower tip or pole of the kneecap. The smaller the A-angle, the more the kneecap is vertically aligned in relation to the tibial tubercle.

The knee has to co-ordinate with the joints of the foot, ankle and hip in normal movements involving the leg, and each of these joints exerts an influence on the knee. In females, the hips may be set wide apart, so the thigh-bones are more diagonal than vertical if you stand with your legs straight and knees close together. If the foot has a flattened arch, or tends to roll inwards excessively into over-pronation, the knee too may be drawn inwards, contributing to knock-knee, which is technically called

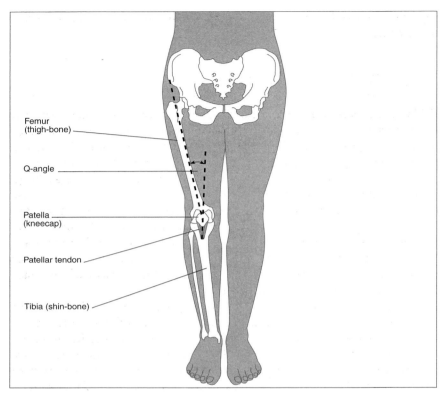

Femur
(thigh-bone)

Q-angle

Patella
(kneecap)

Patellar tendon

Tibia (shin-bone)

The 'Q-angle'

genu valgum. A tendency for the hip to turn inwards has a similar effect. A high-arched foot which tends to roll outwards into over-supination, and a hip which turns outwards, can both contribute to bow leg, or genu varum. A stiff ankle can cause increased mobility in the knee as a compensatory mechanism, but it might instead restrict the movements of all the related joints in the leg. If the hamstrings are especially short or tight, or in cases of degeneration or osteoarthritis of the joint, the knee can be pulled into a bent position, which is called fixed flexion deformity if it is noticeable and cannot be corrected. When the knee curves backwards, or hyperextends, as seen from the side, it is called genu recurvatum, and this is usually associated with excessive flexibility in the tendons at the back of the knee and perhaps weakness in the vastus medialis obliquus part of the quadriceps muscle group. A high kneecap, or patella alta, is often associated with a hyperextending knee. If the kneecap is drawn downwards to be abnormally low in relation to the knee joint, it is called a patella baja, and it is always associated with tightness at the front of the knee and a disruption of normal knee movements.

THE BONES OF THE KNEE

The main part of the knee, the tibiofemoral joint, is formed between the ends of the thigh-bone and the shin-bone. The rounded knuckles of the thigh-bone are called condyles, and their asymmetrical shape dictates the way in which the knee moves. The top of the shin-bone is flattened, so although it is the receiving surface for the thigh-bone condyles, the bones do not fit into each other directly. They are closest together when the knee is straightened fully. This arrangement allows the knee joint greater overall freedom of movement than would otherwise be the case. The bone surfaces are matched to each other, in that the outer (lateral) part of the tibial surface is smaller and rounder than the inner (medial) section, reflecting the relative sizes of the surfaces of the inner (medial) and outer (lateral) femoral condyles.

While the parts of the bones which glide across each other are normally smooth, there are roughened and sometimes slightly raised parts where soft tissues like ligaments and tendons are attached. Right across the middle of the upper surface of the shin-bone, in the front–back (antero-posterior) direction, are the attachment points for the cruciate ligaments and the semilunar cartilages. Just below the top of the front of the shin-bone is a small knob called the tibial tubercle, which is the attachment point of the patellar tendon. At the sides of the thigh-bone and shin-bone are the attachment areas for the inner (medial) and outer (lateral) ligaments.

The kneecap (patellofemoral) joint links the kneecap to the condyles of the thigh-bone. The kneecap is the largest of the body's free-floating bones, technically called sesamoids. Its triangular shape, with the apex downwards, can be seen and felt clearly over the front of the knee. The patellar tendon is attached to its lower tip (pole).

The back of the kneecap is divided into two by a central vertical ridge which allows the bone to fit neatly into the dip between the thigh-bone condyles, although the surfaces of the bones are not shaped to match totally. There are also other ridges, vertical and horizontal, on the back of the kneecap, which mark out the different areas of the bone. When you are standing up and relaxed, the kneecap is not in direct contact with the thigh-bone. When you contract your muscles to straighten and bend your knee, the kneecap is drawn into closer contact with the thigh-bone. Different parts of the kneecap contact the thigh-bone at different stages of the movements, and this pattern varies according to the alignment or position of the kneecap and the efficiency of the muscles which control it.

The bone surfaces within the knee are covered with articular hyaline cartilage, a special cell structure which is smooth, pale, rather glossy and slightly elastic. It serves the important purpose of providing smooth surfaces which, when normally lubricated by synovial fluid, allow for almost friction-free movement, and absorb the compressive forces which the joint might be subjected to, for instance as it bears your weight. This

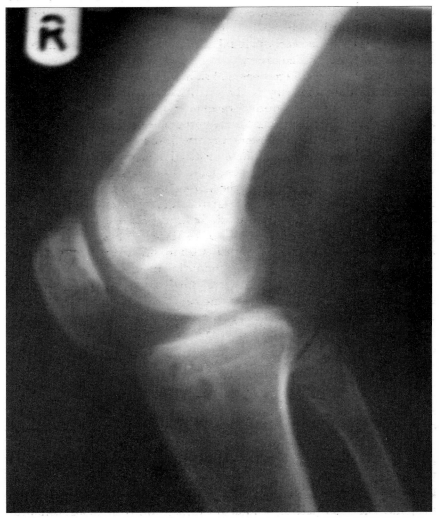

X-ray showing the knee bones

type of cartilage, which adheres closely to the bone ends, must not be confused with the semilunar cartilages, technically called menisci, which are familiar because of the frequency with which they are injured, especially among soccer players and American footballers.

How the bones develop

All the body's bones develop in stages. The process through which a bone develops from its softer cartilage version to the hardened complete shape is called ossification. Most bones consist of separate parts at first, which develop from ossification centres, and grow to meet their adjoining parts at junctions called physes or growth plates, also known as epiphyseal plates. When a bone reaches its full size and shape, the growth plate hardens in a process called fusion.

Long bones like the thigh-bone and shin-bone are already beginning to form when the unborn baby is about ten weeks old. At birth, the main part of the thigh-bone is already formed in miniature, and there is already a secondary ossification centre for the formation of the condyles, just as there is also a secondary ossification centre at the upper end of the shin-bone. The early appearance of these ossification centres in the two bones which form the knee is unique in the body. Fusion of the lower end of the thigh-bone and the upper end of the shin-bone on to the main shafts of their respective bones takes place at the ages of roughly 15 to 17 in females, 17 to 19 in males. In the shin-bone, an extension of the growth plate appears at about the age of 10, to form the basis for the tibial tuberosity, and a secondary ossification centre for it usually develops at about 12 and quickly fuses with the underlying bone.

The kneecap is made up of several small parts whose ossification centres develop somewhere between the ages of 2 and 5 and quickly join together. Ossification centres for the three 'corners' at the edges of the bone appear later on and then fuse with the central part to form the complete bone.

THE SEMILUNAR CARTILAGES

The semilunar cartilages, or menisci, are crescent-shaped soft cushioning buffers which lie over the top of the shin-bone. The inner (medial) one is semicircular, and is attached not only to the shin-bone, but also to the joint capsule and medial ligament at the inner side of the knee, and the transverse ligament (which not everyone has) at the front of the joint. The outer (lateral) semilunar cartilage forms an almost complete circle, and is attached to the shin-bone in between the attachments of the medial semilunar cartilage. At the front, it also bonds with the anterior cruciate ligament, while its back part is attached to the thigh-bone by one or two special meniscofemoral ligaments, and to the popliteus tendon which crosses the back of the knee. Because of the differences in their attachments, the lateral cartilage is much more mobile than the medial.

The blood supply to the semilunar cartilages comes through blood vessels along the outer edges of each, reaching up to about a third of the width of the medial cartilage, and only a quarter of the width of the lateral cartilage. The inner edges of the cartilages do not have a blood supply, so they are technically avascular. The area which receives a blood supply decreases significantly with age. It has been calculated that while about 50 per cent of the outer areas of the cartilages have a blood supply in the newborn child, the area decreases to about 20 per cent by the age of 40. The nerve supply for the cartilages is especially rich at the attachment areas (horns), but totally absent in the middle sections. The sensory nerves at the attachments are thought to have a proprioceptive role, giving information about the knee joint's position.

The semilunar cartilages are made of fibrocartilage, and consist mainly of collagen fibres which are arranged in such a way as to dissipate vertical compressive loading. From the time of birth up to the age of 30, the collagen content of the cartilages increases, and normally does not change until after the age of about 70. Load transmission is considered to be a vital function of the semilunar cartilages: it has been calculated that 50 per cent of the knee's compressive loading is taken through the cartilages when the knee is straight, and up to 85 per cent when the knee is bent to a right angle.

The cartilages also have an important cushioning role in shock absorption, and by absorbing energy they help to protect the underlying articular cartilage and bone structure. They help to make the knee stable, because they are shaped to make the bone surfaces better matched, and because during knee movement they limit extreme motion in any direction. The semilunar cartilages are drawn forwards as you straighten your knee, and their front edges (anterior horns) help to stop the knee from going too far into hyperextension. Similarly, the cartilages are drawn backwards when you bend your knee, and the hind parts (posterior horns) help to limit any abnormal or excessive flexion. Joint nutrition is another function served by the semilunar cartilages. When you are taking weight through your leg, the cartilages help to press the knee joint's synovial fluid into the articular cartilage over the top of the shin-bone.

THE JOINT CAPSULE, LIGAMENTS AND SYNOVIAL LINING

A joint capsule is a kind of enclosing bag of fibrous tissue which surrounds the bones and other joint structures. In the knee, the capsule surrounds the sides and back of the joint, but does not cover the kneecap. Instead, it is blended into the retinacula which are attached to the sides of the kneecap.

Ligaments are thickened bands of connective tissue designed to prevent abnormal movements in a joint. Some ligaments are thickenings of the joint capsule, while others are formed independently of the capsule. Ligaments are only slightly elastic, and they are tight at the natural limit of a joint's movement. In the normal way they protect the joint, and are in turn protected by the reflex contraction of the muscles around them if the joint is put under excessive pressure.

The inner side of the knee is protected by the medial ligament, or tibial collateral ligament, a strong band which links the inner side of the thigh-bone to the shin-bone, and is usually attached to the inner (medial) semilunar cartilage and the joint capsule. The medial ligament protects the knee when it is put under any stress which threatens to open up the inner side of the joint, as in falling on to that side of the leg with the foot sliding sideways away from the body, or doing the splits sideways and having an unexpected or excessive force push down from the other side of the knee. The lateral or fibular collateral ligament is attached to the thigh-bone and the head of the fibula on the outer side of the knee. It usually blends with the biceps femoris tendon, but has no attachment to the lateral semilunar cartilage. It protects the knee against pressures on the outer side of the joint. The back of the knee is protected by the oblique and arcuate popliteal ligaments, which are both blended with the joint capsule. Although they are relatively weak, they help protect against stresses which would over-stretch the back of the knee into hyperextension.

Right in the centre of the knee are the two cruciate ligaments. The anterior cruciate ligament is attached near the centre of the top of the shin-bone, joining the front part of the outer semilunar cartilage, and spreads upwards and outwards to its attachment on the inner part of the outer (lateral) thigh-bone condyle. The posterior cruciate ligament is shorter, stronger, and more vertically aligned. It lies behind the anterior cruciate on the shin-bone, is attached to the back part of the outer semilunar cartilage, and extends upwards and inwards to be attached to the innermost edge of the inner (medial) condyle.

As in all moving joints, the knee-joint capsule is lined with a synovial membrane which produces synovial fluid, a yellowish, viscous lubricant for the joint, which also helps to provide nutrition for the articular cartilage and to remove any unwanted matter. The synovial membrane forms folds and fringes in the joint, which fill in irregular spaces within the joint.

Fat pads are accumulations of fatty (adipose) tissue in the synovial membrane. At the front of the knee, the infrapatellar fat pad lies between the synovial membrane and the patellar tendon, and the membrane goes round the fat pad to form the so-called alar folds which protrude backwards into the knee joint. Over the top of the kneecap it forms a large pouch of synovial fluid called the suprapatellar bursa, which lies between the quadriceps tendon and the thigh-bone. There are many other bursae around the knee to provide friction-free movement, including the prepatellar bursa over the lower part of the kneecap under the skin, the infrapatellar bursa between the tibial tubercle and the skin, the deep infrapatellar bursa between the shin-bone and the patellar tendon, and numerous bursae which separate the ligaments and tendons on either side of the knee from each other and from any structures which might rub against them.

The knee's muscles and tendons

The knee is surrounded by extremely strong muscles whose interplay gives co-ordinated movement and stability to the joint. The muscles on the front of the thigh are the knee extensors, which straighten the knee, those at the back are the flexors which bend it, the adductors along the inner thigh draw the leg inwards, and the outer side of the knee is stabilized by the iliotibial tract, which links to the major hip muscles.

Muscles on the front of the thigh

The quadriceps femoris muscle group is the large mass of muscle on the front of the thigh that crosses the front of the knee to be attached to the tibial tubercle on the shin-bone by the patellar tendon, whose technical name is ligamentum patellae. Three parts of the quadriceps group, the outer vastus lateralis, central vastus intermedius and inner vastus medialis, are attached to the thigh and only cross the knee. The longest section, rectus femoris, is a two-joint muscle attached to the front of the pelvic bone, which crosses both the hip and the knee. All four parts are joined into the quadriceps tendon which is bonded to the upper edge of the kneecap at the lower end of the thigh. The kneecap is sited inside the

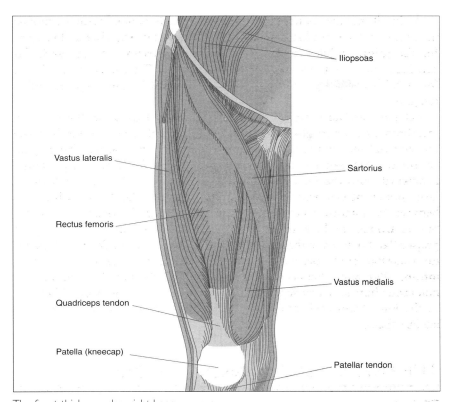

Iliopsoas

Vastus lateralis

Sartorius

Rectus femoris

Vastus medialis

Quadriceps tendon

Patella (kneecap)

Patellar tendon

The front-thigh muscles, right knee

quadriceps tendon, and anchored on either side by expansions called retinacula which come from the outer and inner quadriceps muscles.

The quadriceps group straightens the knee against gravity or a resistance, as in leg extension exercises or kicking. Rectus femoris also helps to bend the hip against gravity, working with iliopsoas, the hip flexor muscles. The quadriceps muscles have to pay out, contracting eccentrically, when you bend your knee under the influence of gravity, as in going down stairs or squatting. When you stand still with your legs relaxed there is little demand on the quadriceps muscles, even though the body's weight is transmitted slightly in front of the knees, as the knee ligaments are efficient enough to prevent overbalancing. In walking, running, jumping and hopping, the quadriceps play an important propulsive role.

Over the top of the quadriceps group lies the sartorius muscle, the longest in the body, which stretches from the top of the front of the pelvic bone to the inner side of the top of the shin-bone. It helps to bend the hip

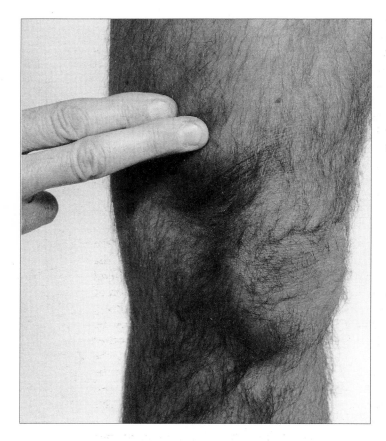

The vastus medialis obliquus muscle, left knee

and knee, and to lift and turn the thigh outwards from the hip (technically into abduction and lateral rotation). Under the lower part of the quadriceps group is a tiny muscle, articularis genus, which serves to pull the synovial bursa above the kneecap upwards when you straighten your knee.

Vastus medialis obliquus (VMO)

Of the knee's controlling muscles, the vastus medialis was defined as the 'key to the knee' many years ago by eminent orthopaedic surgeon Mr Smillie. This muscle forms the inner (medial) part of the quadriceps muscle group, and is divided into two: a longer section sited more or less vertically along the inner thigh, and a shorter, more diagonally orientated part. Mr Smillie and many others have highlighted the importance of this lower part of the muscle, which is called vastus medialis obliquus (VMO). This element has an action potential count which is twice as great as the other components of the quadriceps group, and it has to exert 60 per cent more force to lock the knee during the last 15 degrees of full knee extension than the rest of the extensor muscles apply to straighten the knee from the bent position up to that angle. The VMO has the special function of holding the kneecap steady in its groove on the thigh-bone, as it is the only muscle attached to the kneecap from the inner side.

Certain sports, such as squash, fencing and wicket-keeping in cricket, tend to undermine the VMO, because they involve too much weightbearing over the bent knee without enough knee-straightening movements. Conversely, sports which involve reaching up, jumping or kicking, such as tennis, badminton, basketball, soccer, rugby and American football, tend to create strong VMO muscles.

Muscles of the inner thigh

Five muscles link the inner thigh to the pelvic bone. The smallest is the pectineus, which is a flat muscle in the groin region at the top of the thigh. The three adductor muscles, longus, magnus and brevis, extend along the inner side of the thigh-bone from the pelvic bone. The tendon of adductor longus is easy to feel in the groin region when you are sitting down, especially if you tense it by pressing the thigh inwards towards the other leg. Gracilis is a long thin muscle which lies on top of the other inner thigh muscles, and stretches from the pelvic bone to just below the inner side of the knee, so it acts on both the hip and the knee. At the attachment below the knee it joins the tendons of sartorius and semitendinosus to form a structure called the 'pes anserinus' (goose's foot), which curves round the top inner edge of the shin-bone.

With pectineus, the adductor muscles draw the thigh inwards against gravity or a resistance. They are of primary importance for kicking the football in soccer, for instance. Depending on the position of the leg, each can be active during other hip movements, including inward (medial) rotation, flexion and extension. Gracilis helps to flex the hip and knee, and to turn them inwards, as well as helping to draw the thigh in towards the other leg.

The inner thigh muscles co-ordinate with the other muscles controlling the thigh and knee. They come into play especially when the front-thigh muscles are working under pressure: if you are pushing very heavy weights on a leg press machine you may turn your legs inwards, bringing your knees together, in order to recruit the adductors to help the front-thigh muscles. A tendency to run with the legs turned in and heels kicking out, using the adductors more than normal, is a sure sign of over-training or lack of fitness in the child or teenage runner.

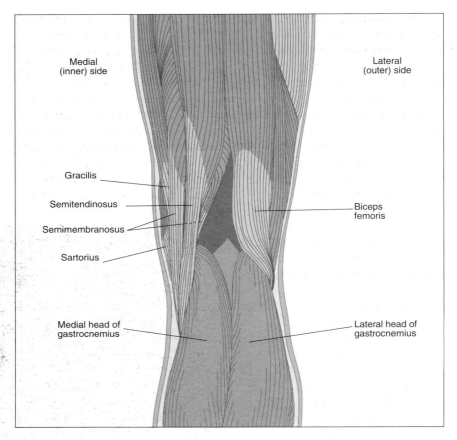

Medial
(inner) side

Lateral
(outer) side

Gracilis

Semitendinosus

Semimembranosus

Sartorius

Biceps
femoris

Medial head of
gastrocnemius

Lateral head of
gastrocnemius

The muscles and tendons at the back of the right knee

Muscles and tendons at the back of the knee

The three hamstring muscles at the back of the thigh extend from the seat-bone (ischial tuberosity) to just below the back of the knee. Biceps femoris is attached to the head of the fibula and the outer part of the shin-bone, while semimembranosus and semitendinosus are joined to the top of the shin-bone at the inner side of the knee. Semitendinosus forms part of the pes anserinus with sartorius and gracilis. You can feel the cords of the semitendinosus and gracilis tendons behind the inner part of your knee when you sit with the joint bent and your foot turned slightly inwards. Semitendinosus is the more prominent. Semimembranosus lies more deeply, and so is harder to feel. On the outer side, the biceps femoris tendon is easy to feel when you bend your knee and turn your foot slightly outwards.

The hamstrings extend the thigh backwards at the hip and bend the knee. Being two-joint muscles with very long tendons, they are relatively easily injured through explosive sports like sprinting, especially because they normally only have about 60–70 per cent of the strength of the quadriceps muscles. Cyclists develop very strong hamstrings which can be roughly equal in strength to their quadriceps muscles. The hamstrings tend to become tight through over-activity or during childhood and teenage growth spurts. When they are shortened, they pull the knee into the bent position and the pelvis backwards. In older age, the combination of joint degeneration and shortened hamstrings tends to hold the knee in fixed flexion deformity. The abnormal position is called a contracture.

The popliteus muscle is situated inside the back of the knee. It extends from the outer side of the thigh-bone condyle downwards and inwards to the top of the shin-bone. It is connected to the arcuate ligament, joint capsule and the outer semilunar cartilage, and probably acts to pull the cartilage backwards when the knee is bent and the thigh-bone twisted outwards. Popliteus helps to turn your shin-bone inwards when your foot is not fixed. Its main function is probably to unlock the knee to let it bend after it has been straightened out fully.

The gastrocnemius muscle forms the bulky part of the calf and, with the underlying soleus muscle, ends in the Achilles tendon which is attached to the heel-bone. Whereas soleus joins on to the shin-bone, gastrocnemius is attached to the thigh-bone above the knee by two strong tendons joined on to the condyles. The two heads of the muscle also attach to the capsule of the knee joint. You can feel and see them behind the knee, especially if you stand on your toes and bend the knee slightly. Underneath the

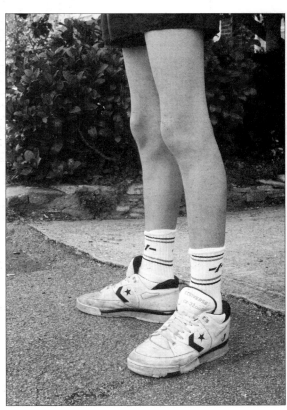

A teenage growth spurt can tighten the hamstrings and draw the knees into a slightly bent position

outer (lateral) head of gastrocnemius lies another muscle, plantaris.

The main action of these calf muscles is to point the toes downwards against gravity, so they provide the main impetus when you go up on to your toes, or push off your toes during walking, running, jumping, hopping or skipping. Because gastrocnemius is attached above the knee, it also comes into play when you bend your knee hard against a heavy resistance. If there is weakness in the hamstring muscles, the calf muscles on the same side usually compensate for it, and vice versa. If soleus is especially weak, you will find it difficult to go up on your toes while keeping your knee straight. If you have limped for any length of time, the calf muscles weaken, and you may develop a habit of walking flat-footed without lifting your heel off the ground at the right time, which may make you turn your leg outwards from the hip. This abnormal gait pattern can create extra jarring and shearing pressures on the knee, which can cause pain or prolong a knee problem if that caused the limp in the first place.

The iliotibial tract (band) at the outer side of the knee

The iliotibial tract is a strong band formed from the fascia lata, the covering sac of tissue which holds the thigh muscles in place. You can see the iliotibial tract clearly on the outer side of your thigh, especially on the lower part, when you straighten your knee hard. It is attached to the upper outer edge of the shin-bone and the top of the fibula, and is controlled by a muscle called tensor fasciae latae, which links the pelvic bone to the upper part of the iliotibial tract. The main seat muscle, gluteus maximus, which forms the curve of your bottom, is also attached to the iliotibial tract and acts on it to help hold the thigh-bone in a stable position relative to the shin-bone when the front-thigh muscles are relaxed.

The gluteus maximus and the iliotibial tract system tend to become very strong and well-defined through sports which involve running, bending and turning, like field hockey, rugby and squash, and through activities involving outward hip movements, as in classical ballet and the different forms of karate.

Knee pain and other symptoms

4

Technically, the objective factors which are the evidence of an injury or physical problem are called clinical signs. Clinical signs can be seen, felt or sometimes heard on a physical examination of the area and related parts, or they show up through diagnostic tests, such as X-rays, scans, arthrograms or blood tests. Symptoms are the sensations you feel which make you aware that something is wrong. There is usually an overlap between signs and symptoms, in that some of the sensations you feel from the inside are caused by factors which can be seen and felt externally by the practitioner. In any kind of knee problem, the three main signs and symptoms which you are likely to notice are pain, swelling and functional impairment, although you may also notice others, such as changes in the skin colour, temperature or sensitivity.

KNEE PAIN

Pain, technically known as nociception, is a perception of discomfort, an internal awareness of an unpleasant sensation. The way in which the body's nervous system reacts to unpleasant stimuli such as tissue damage through injury or inflammation is very complex, and not yet fully understood. It is known that special nerves called nociceptors pick up the sensations of excessive mechanical pressure or heat and transmit signals to the spinal cord, which may react by setting up some kind of protective strategy for the painful tissues. There are probably different mechanisms governing acute pain in an immediate injury and chronic pain relating to the longer-term after-effects of an injury, inflammation or disease. In inflammation and chronic pain, more nerves become sensitive and transmit pain signals due to chemical changes, and the balance between the sensation nerves which transmit the pain messages and the inhibitory nerves which would normally damp down that message system is altered.

Pain is a subjective symptom which varies according to the individual. Only you can know what kind of pain you feel and how much it hurts. People with a so-called high pain threshold can bear a lot of pain apparently easily. Perhaps in some cases they do not feel pain in situations where other people might. A low pain threshold means a very acute awareness of pain, possibly in some cases unreasonably and to an exaggerated degree. While other people may be able to offer sympathy and understanding of your pain, no one can share it with you. It is also extremely difficult to compare your experience of pain with someone else's, even if the circumstances appear similar.

Pain patterns

Knee pain can not only be caused by injury, but can also result from infection, inflammation or disease. In different conditions, there can be pain in almost any situation: during activities, on certain movements, at rest, when still, or in bed at night. Pain in itself is often an imprecise guide as to what has gone wrong with the knee. The amount of pain you feel is not necessarily directly proportional to what is wrong. This is one of several reasons why you should not try to diagnose your problem by yourself. You may think you know exactly where your pain is, but in fact it is unlikely that you can localize it accurately. The nerve systems in the knee are arranged in a complicated way. The place where you perceive your knee pain is not necessarily its source, as knee pain may in fact be transferred from a related region, especially the hip, or sometimes the lower back. Pain transferred through the nerve systems from the real problem area to an unrelated part further away is called referred pain. The actual problem which causes the pain transfer is often called a 'trapped nerve', which is a popular descriptive term rather than a technical one.

In the immediate stage of a traumatic injury, the pain can be very severe or surprisingly mild. The pain associated with complex damage caused by twisting, shearing or direct trauma can be excruciating. If you twist your knee badly, you may feel a sickening sensation as if your leg has been cut in half at the knee. There may be immediate pain, but sometimes the knee feels better straight away if you manage to get it moving gently without placing your weight on it. Even a major injury, such as a tear in the anterior cruciate ligament, can happen without much immediate pain. A footballer in this situation often tries to play on, only to find that the knee gives way and becomes painful because of the functional deficit.

Overuse injuries usually start with just a slight pain during or after a repetitive activity like running, and the pain increases gradually over a space of time if you keep on aggravating the injury. Sometimes the pain can become extremely severe if you injure the weakened joint further, or if food intolerance superimposes additional pain.

According to the nature of your problem, you may feel generalized pain, apparently spread over the whole knee joint, or localized pain which is confined to a precise spot or area. If any part of your knee is painful or sensitive on direct pressure, it is described as tender, or tender to touch. Pain can be consistent, or it may seem to move around the knee in a haphazard fashion. Your pain may be directly related to certain leg movements or positions. It can occur at rest. If you feel pain in bed at night, it may happen when your leg is still, or because one knee is pressing against the other, or because you have moved to turn over. Your pain may be worst in the morning, later on during the day, or at night.

Every pain has its own characteristic nature. If your pain is fairly constant, and present most or all of the time at a relatively low level, you might describe it as 'nagging', or 'like a toothache'. Pain may be intermittent, occasional, frequent or persistent; slight or agonizing. It may appear to occur, disappear and recur in an arbitrary way, or there may be a recognizable pattern to it. There may be a cycle of pain, or a process of development. For instance, a sharp pain which comes on suddenly usually settles to a duller level after the first few days, and may subside to a background dull ache if it lasts longer. The way in which a pain behaves, even when it appears arbitrary, is called the pain pattern. It is a vital guide for diagnosis in many knee problems, and is always significant in the assessment of functional impairment.

Pain in its earliest stage is described as acute; after the first few days as subacute or recent. If it lasts for more than a couple of weeks, up to months or years, it is described as chronic. Sometimes people use the terms 'acute' and 'chronic' to describe a high level or degree of pain, but they are probably more accurately used as an expression of the time during which a pain has been present.

Fear, stress and pain

Because it is a subjective symptom, pain is always 'psychological', or at least influenced by your state of mind and mental well-being. This is not the same as saying that you are imagining your pain and if you pull yourself together the pain will go away. Pain is always real to the person experiencing it.

Fear and stress have a significant influence on knee pain. They can make an existing pain worse, or they can actually cause pain, although this is rare. There is no doubt that fear and stress hinder recovery from any kind of knee problem.

Fear can play a big part in your perception of pain. The fact that your knee hurts can be a frightening experience, especially if you do not understand fully why it is painful, or if you have never felt similar pain before. Fear focuses your mind more intensely on the pain and makes you guard the knee by avoiding using it normally and by holding it stiffly. A vicious circle is set up which makes the pain more intense, so that it dominates your mind and makes you protect the knee even more.

Stress, in the sense of excessive pressure which causes tension and over-anxiety, can affect your physical and mental well-being. It can have a negative effect on very young children, adults, older age groups, and on males and females alike. Most people have to cope with some level of this type of stress. Children may be over-pressurized, for instance, through parental expectations, sibling rivalry, peer group competitiveness or examinations. Adults can be stressed by family or emotional problems, or difficult working conditions. The combination of too little time, too much work, too many obligations, too much tiredness and too little energy to get everything done can be seriously undermining.

Stress can undermine many aspects of your normal body functioning, and so contribute to joint pain, including knee pain. It can be a factor in different kinds of illness, especially for instance glandular fever, myalgic encephalomyelitis and irritable bowel syndrome. Stress can interfere with sleep, reducing your energy levels through fatigue. It can impair your judgement, and make you unreasonably irritable or fearful. It can cause muscular tightness or spasm, undermining your posture as well as your ability to move your joints freely and fluently.

Depression or low mood can have an effect on knee pain. When the

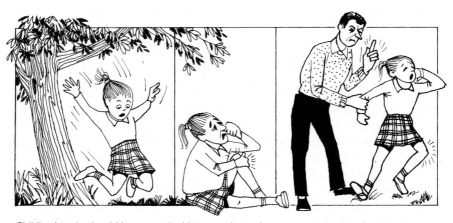

Children's pain should be treated with sympathy and care, not anger, no matter what the cause

symptoms of depression are severe enough, the body's muscles lose their normal tone. This means that the natural tension in the muscles which prepares them for contraction and activity is weakened, the muscles become soft and flabby, and their energy is undermined. This adds to the depressed person's feelings of unnatural listlessness and fatigue. It also means that the knees gain less protection from their stabilizing muscles, which increases the functional problems associated with any problems in one or both knee joints.

Psychosomatic pain

Very rarely, there is no physical cause to explain the patient's complaint of pain, so the assumption has to be that the pain is psychosomatic, and is caused by psychological or emotional factors. This conclusion can only be reached after all possible tests and investigations have been applied and the results found to be normal. It is a situation which requires great sensitivity on the part of the practitioners involved. The patient will feel insecure or resentful if any practitioner lets slip careless comments which reveal indifference or irritation towards the patient's pain. Making the patient feel undermined or misunderstood will not help him or her to get better. Every practitioner involved in the case has to be totally supportive, to build up the patient's confidence that the solution to the problem of the pain and its underlying causes can be found.

KNEE SWELLING

Swelling (effusion) in the knee means that there is extra fluid within the joint, and it is a sure sign that there is something wrong. A traumatic injury involving shearing, wrenching or jarring movements usually causes swelling in the knee. This means that there is damage to one or more of the joint structures. The damage may involve the synovial lining and joint capsule, blood vessels, any of the knee's ligaments, the cartilages (menisci) or the bones and their covering of articular cartilage. When injury-induced swelling is present, the joint usually also feels warm to the touch, although the practitioner may feel this temperature difference more easily than the injured person. The skin over the joint may be normal or it may appear shiny, especially if the effusion is large. In a traumatic injury or after an operation, visible bruising may accompany the swelling.

The swelling may consist of synovial fluid, the liquid formed in the joint's synovial lining, which bathes the bone surfaces to allow friction-free movement. In this case, it is called a traumatic synovitis, and the fluid is light yellow, often described as straw-coloured. This type of swelling

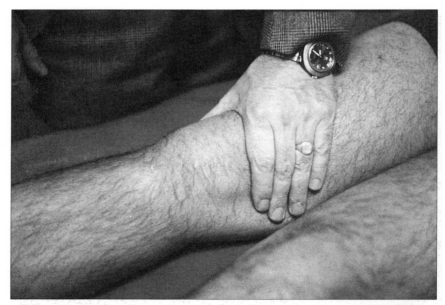

Swelling caused by internal damage can be slight, like this small effusion by the practitioner's index finger

may not appear until several hours after the injury, and it indicates that, whatever else has been damaged, no internal blood vessels are involved.

A bad injury may cause bleeding inside the joint. Blood which fills a joint is technically called a haemarthrosis. Sometimes, a haemarthrosis can occur as a complication following an operation. Severe trauma to the knee can result in the joint being completely filled with blood, so that the fluid is wholly red. If there is only minor internal bleeding, the fluid is yellow coloured with red streaks in it. A haemarthrosis usually comes up as immediate swelling, and indicates that blood vessels have been torn.

The swelling in an injured knee can be large or small, sometimes so small that it is almost imperceptible. It can appear over the whole joint, including the back of the knee, or it can be isolated to a small patch on one side or the other. The amount of swelling does not necessarily correlate with the severity of the injury: a trivial knock can result in enormous swelling, while total rupture of a key ligament like the anterior cruciate very often only causes a minute effusion.

Overuse injuries can also cause swelling in the knee, but it is usually limited. If the swelling is large, especially if it feels hot, it is likely to have some other cause apart from the overuse injury, which might be disease, infection, an inflammatory condition or food intolerance.

Swelling is an important feature of most diseases which affect joints,

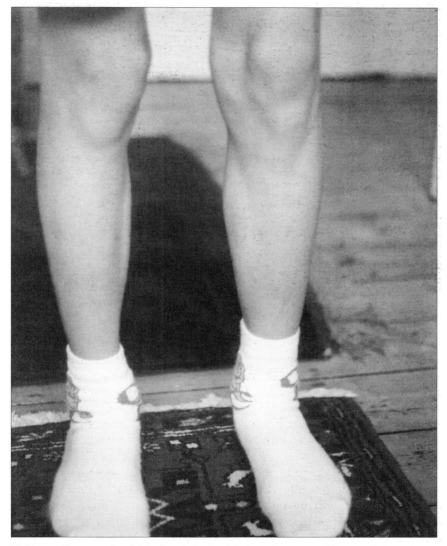

Visible swelling over the tibial tubercle in the right knee in a case of Osgood-Schlatter's condition

such as rheumatoid arthritis and tuberculosis. When the disease is active, the affected joints often feel very hot, both from the inside and externally to the touch. It is also common for the skin to be reddened and shiny-looking. Confusingly, similar signs and symptoms can appear if you have food intolerance reactions.

Knee swelling can damage the joint's articular surfaces and inhibit the nerves controlling the joint (mechanoreceptors), which causes the muscles to stop working properly. The longer the knee is allowed to remain swollen, the more damaging these effects are, so knee swelling should never be ignored.

SUPPLEMENTARY CAUSES OF KNEE PAIN

Food intolerance

Reactions to irritant foods and drinks can be a cause of knee pain, swelling and other symptoms. It is often difficult for people to accept that food intolerance might play a part in their knee problem. Food intolerance, unlike allergy, is not a specific reaction to a specific substance. Very often the food or drink involved does not seem 'unhealthy' in itself, and it can be something that is taken regularly without problems in the normal way. The reaction can happen with almost anything that you might eat or drink, and is especially likely to relate to things that you take in habitually every day.

Food intolerance can affect anyone at any age. I have known a two-year-old child whose foot became too hot and painful to walk on as a result of eating oranges. There are certain defined situations in which food intolerance reactions are likely to occur. You become more vulnerable to food intolerance if you are run-down, over-tired, over-anxious, ill, suffering from an infection, or in the grip of stress or emotional distress. Food intolerance often follows a stomach upset or an episode of irritable bowel syndrome. You can become sensitive to almost any food or drink if you have it every day, for instance if you drink lots of coffee, or if you suddenly start eating large quantities of a fruit which has come into season. One of my patients became intolerant to lettuce, which she did not like particularly, but which she ate every day because she thought it was good for her. Another reacted to peas, which she ate frequently because she loved them. Although literally anything can become an irritant, certain foods and drinks are more likely to cause reactions in a sensitive person. These include chocolate, oranges, nectarines, tomatoes, tomato sauce or paste, strawberries, dairy products, spicy foods (especially curries), wheat, seafood, pork, fizzy drinks (especially the so-called 'diet' versions), alcohol, tea, coffee, juices, preservatives and colourings.

Food Intolerance

Reactions
- headaches
- skin blemishes
- nausea
- vomiting
- joint pain
- heat
- swelling
- stiffness

Reasons
- excessive intake of irritant foods or drinks
- frequent intake of one type of food or drink
- increased sensitivity due to: *illness*
  infections
  fatigue
  stress
  stomach upsets
  injury

Cure
- diary recording: *food and drink intake*
  activities
  feelings
  reactions

- rest, relaxation and stress reduction
- elimination of suspect foods and drinks
- regular, well-balanced diet
- plenty of green vegetables
- regular plentiful water throughout the day

Effects of food intolerance

Food intolerance can cause headaches, nausea, vomiting, skin blemishes, joint pains, stiffness or swelling. The reaction can happen within an hour of eating or drinking the irritant, or much later. In the case of wheat, the reaction can be delayed for a couple of days. The symptoms may be very mild at first, but they quickly build up to a very severe degree. If your diet is varied, and you do not eat or drink the irritant again, the pain and other symptoms usually ease of their own accord within a few days. Otherwise the symptoms will last.

When food intolerance affects the knee, the typical feature is that the joint swells up and/or becomes very stiff for no apparent reason. The skin over the knee may be reddened and shiny, and the joint usually feels warm or even hot, both internally and if you touch the surface. Although in some cases there is marked swelling and stiffness but little pain, in others the pain can be excruciatingly intense, and will not be relieved by cold applications or painkillers. The effect can be alarming, because it may seem that something terrible has happened. Where the food intolerance reaction is the primary problem in the knee, the symptoms appear to happen out of the blue. Secondary to an operation, injury or other knee problem, the food intolerance reactions are superimposed on the original symptoms.

Food intolerance can be very confusing for the patient. If there is any doubt as to what is causing the new symptoms, the doctor will screen the patient to exclude alternative possibilities. Food intolerance can also be depressing, if it means that the patient has to be deprived of a favourite food or drink. Fortunately, the reactions are usually temporary, so elimination of the irritant is necessary only while the knee is symptomatic and the patient vulnerable.

Controlling food intolerance

If you have symptoms which might be due to food intolerance, you need to keep a diary of your symptoms in relation to your activities and your food and drink intake. The diary should include an accurate record of how much plain water you drink each day. Try to drink at least one glass of water whenever you eat food or drink other types of fluid. You should aim at ten full glasses of water at least. Children dehydrate more quickly than adults, so it is especially important to make sure that they acquire the good habit of drinking plenty of plain water every day.

As a precaution, you should eliminate any likely irritants which are not nutritionally essential, such as chocolates, spicy foods, fizzy drinks, juices, alcohol, tea and coffee. Avoid convenience foods. Eat regular well-balanced meals, including plenty of green vegetables. You should also try

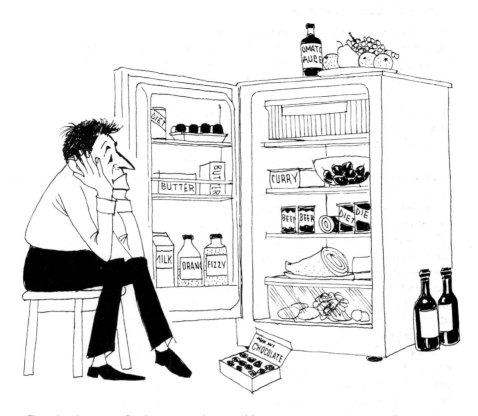

Choosing the wrong foods can cause knee problems

to reduce known stresses and avoid fatigue. If you can, you should rest, preferably lying down, for at least ten minutes during each day. If you are very tense and pressured, it may help you to learn and practise relaxation techniques, or to have treatment from a professional counsellor, psychologist or psychotherapist.

Once the food intolerance reactions have been controlled, you can gradually re-introduce some of the eliminated foods and drinks, if you wish. Watch out for adverse reactions, so that you can quickly cut out any substances to which you are still sensitive.

Reflex sympathetic dystrophy

Reflex sympathetic dystrophy (RSD) can be an important factor in knee problems. Also known as Sudeck's atrophy or causalgia, it is an unusual condition which can cause very severe pain and disability. It is considered rare, but may be more common than people think, because it is often missed, ignored or mis-diagnosed. It can happen in the arm, but is probably more common in the leg. It occurs most often in the lower leg, ankle and foot, but can affect the knee, thigh and hip. Sometimes the condition starts in the foot and spreads upwards to involve the knee. In some cases RSD affects the knee first, and may then spread along the leg.

The effects of RSD

There are several characteristic signs and symptoms of RSD. There is always pain which is not directly related to an injury or tissue damage. The pain is either out of proportion and far greater than would normally be expected, or it does not follow the pattern which would be in keeping with the injury or damage that has occurred. There are changes related to problems with the circulatory system, technically known as vasomotor disturbances, which affect the appearance and feel of the skin. The skin is often extremely sensitive to the touch. It may change colour to be paler, redder or darker than normal. The skin may also feel clammy and slightly sweaty even when the patient is not hot. It may have cool or warm patches. The pulse may be difficult to feel as compared to the sound side. The hairs on the skin tend to thin out or disappear and the growth rate of the nails slows down. A typical feature of RSD is the tendency for the affected area in the leg to turn a deep mottled purple colour when the patient stands up and puts the foot to the floor. The affected area may be swollen, but the muscles are wasted and thin. The affected joints become increasingly stiff and immobile.

How RSD happens

Reflex sympathetic dystrophy can occur after illnesses, operations or injuries, and sometimes it happens for no apparent reason. It may be related to circulatory problems. RSD can happen to anyone, but seems to occur most readily in people who are anxious about their physical problems or have other worries. Patients may be at special risk if they are not used to being ill or injured, would like to understand and control every aspect of their treatment, and find it difficult to trust a practitioner to look after their welfare. Psychological distress is an important feature of the condition. RSD in itself arouses a high level of anxiety, because of the apparently arbitrary nature and severity of the symptoms.

After an injury, the pain of RSD makes itself felt at the time when the patient should in the normal way be feeling better. Typically, as the pain sets in, the patient finds it increasingly difficult to engage in normal levels of physical activities and exercises. Trying to do the same amount of exercise makes the pain worse, never mind trying to do more. In the early stages of RSD, rest for a few days can make the pain reduce, but trying to exercise immediately brings it on again, so the patient naturally tends to do less and less. The pain can interfere with all aspects of normal life, including sleep. Once RSD is established, the pain can be unremitting if it is not treated appropriately. Some patients are diagnosed and treated quickly after the symptoms of RSD first appear. The unlucky ones sometimes wait for years before finding a practitioner who can diagnose the problem correctly and institute the right treatment programme.

How RSD is diagnosed and treated

The first clue to the diagnosis is in the patient's description of the pain and any other noticeable symptoms. When the diagnosis is missed or mistaken, it is usually because the practitioner has no experience of RSD, or is unsympathetic to the patient's pain and believes the description is exaggerated. To confirm the diagnosis, the experienced doctor will first exclude any other possible causes of pain. In RSD, the skin changes, swelling and muscle wasting are seen when the patient is physically examined. A bone scan may show increased activity in the painful area. X-rays may show some degree of osteoporosis. An injection of pain-relieving drug into the lower back to anaesthetize the controlling nerve systems usually produces immediate pain relief which lasts for a couple of days. This technique is called sympathetic blockade, and is used both for diagnosis and for treatment.

Treatments which involve interfering directly with the affected area usually make the pain of RSD worse, so experienced practitioners avoid aggravating it with injections, massage, manipulations, electrotherapy or exercises. Sometimes the first hint that the patient has RSD is a painful reaction to a treatment which never causes pain in normal circumstances. Treatments for RSD are usually applied indirectly. As the pain is so intense, drugs may not help unless they are particularly strong painkillers. Sympathetic blockade is an effective means of pain relief, although the injections into the lower back may have to be repeated many times before the patient stops feeling the pain altogether. Sometimes surgery is used to cut through the controlling nerves to block the pain, usually as a last resort. RSD can also be treated successfully without sympathetic blockade or surgery.

Treating RSD patients is always complex. Physiotherapy techniques are directed at improving function in all the related areas, without disturbing the affected part. The aim is not simply to get the stiff joints moving and strengthen up the wasted muscles, but to revive and normalize the circulatory and nerve systems as the basis for restoring normal joint and muscle function. In the early stages of treatment for RSD involving the

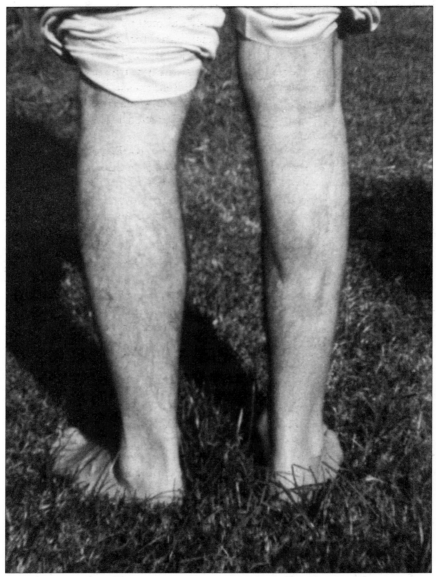

Wasting of the right calf muscles in a case of Reflex Sympathetic Dystrophy

knee, this can mean treating the hip and lower back with mobilizations, massage and perhaps electrical muscle stimulation. I also always treat the upper back and shoulder blade region, as this is almost invariably tight and malfunctioning in RSD patients. Acupuncture to the lower and upper back can be very helpful. Remedial exercises are set for all the painfree parts of the body, so the painful leg is only indirectly involved.

The patient can also be taught to imagine that the affected leg feels the same as the sound one using visualization techniques. It is sometimes easiest to teach these techniques in the warm supportive environment of the hydrotherapy pool, and the patient may find it easier to practise them at home in the comfort of the bath. By mastering visualization techniques the patient can exert some control over the affected leg to the extent of altering its temperature and colour.

Food intolerance is frequently a factor in RSD, so the patient has to be made aware of how to recognize, control and prevent adverse reactions to foods and drinks.

Probably all RSD patients should have some psychological treatment from a psychotherapist, clinical psychologist or counsellor, to deal with stress related to the condition itself as well as any worries or emotional distress that may have preceded it. Many patients find this difficult to accept. Coming to terms with it and learning to trust a suitable practitioner can be important steps towards recovery from RSD.

Fear is the biggest stumbling block to recovery. The patient naturally develops a fear of physical activity, in case a minor over-exertion leads to further intense pain. The patient's confidence has to be built up in conjunction with a very carefully tailored progressive programme of physical activity. The physiotherapist must monitor the exercise programme carefully, and adjust it immediately if even the hint of a problem arises. This control has to be maintained until the patient has fully recovered.

For the majority of RSD patients, treatment may extend over several years. That said, most patients should recover fully or at least to the point where they can do most of what they want, provided the treatment has been accurate and appropriate to their individual needs.

FUNCTIONAL IMPAIRMENT

Functional impairment means the loss of the normal ability to move the knee freely and to control its position. It can be very subtle, to the extent that you may be unaware that your knee is not working properly. At the other extreme, you may be unable to move the knee at all.

Locking

A locked knee is a definite indication of quite serious internal derangement, and it is frightening when it happens. The typical pattern is for the knee to get completely stuck when the joint is at a certain angle, so that you cannot bend or straighten it. In most cases, flicking it gently in a twisting motion will free it. More rarely, the joint cannot be freed by this gentle self-manipulation exercise, although it might gradually regain its freedom of movement if you protect it in a bandage and try to move it gently, day by day. The most common cause of the true locked knee is a tear in one of the soft semilunar cartilages (menisci).

Although the locked knee is a very definite event, there are some instances when the knee seems to get locked, but in fact in a slightly different way from the true locked knee. Pseudo-locking can be caused by poor co-ordination in the kneecap joint, kneecap subluxation, or muscle spasm. It is different from true locking, in that the knee is not completely immobilized, and it can be freed without a twisting manipulation.

Giving way

An injured knee can give way for a variety of reasons, and in different situations. When it gives way completely, you fall over. This means that the knee is grossly unstable, and that the joint's co-ordination is poor. An unstable knee is most likely to give way when it is bent and bearing your bodyweight, as in stepping down a stair or pavement. In some cases, it gives way when there is a twisting motion. More rarely, it can give way during normal walking.

Giving way can be the result of almost any knee problem, including cartilage (meniscus) injuries, bone damage, ligament tears, or kneecap injuries. During the teenage growth spurts, the knees can give way as a result of muscle imbalance or deficit, especially weakness in the front-thigh muscles. In patients of any age, episodes of partial or total giving way, which seem to be caused by a weakness around the knee, can in fact be due to a hip or back problem which has interfered with the nerve control of the leg.

Instead of giving way completely, an injured knee may feel as though it is about to give way, so that you feel unstable or even stumble slightly. This can be caused by a variety of problems. It is a typical feature of the anterior cruciate tear, where you may feel this unsteadiness if you turn slightly to one side while standing up.

Clicking, grating and creaking

Even healthy knees can make loud and alarming noises, especially when they are bent under load, as in going up and down stairs. The most common cause of clicking, grating or creaking emanating from the knee is stiffness in the kneecap (patellofemoral) joint.

If the knee tends to give an isolated click when the joint is held in a certain position, it can be a sign of stiffness in the main knee (tibiofemoral) joint. If the click is painful, it might be a sign of internal damage such as a cartilage (meniscus) tear. Painful clicking can cause inhibition to the knee's controlling muscles, contributing to a cycle of functional impairment.

Co-ordination loss

Any knee injury or condition results in proprioceptive loss, because pain and swelling disrupt the knee's normal nerve mechanisms. Sometimes this is due to direct damage to the nerves through tearing or shearing. It can also be caused by pressure, if there is a lot of blood or synovial or tissue fluid compressing the knee. Because of the proprioceptive loss, there is also a reduction in the joint's kinaesthetic sense, which is the knee's in-built awareness of its position and movement.

The injured knee also suffers a loss of co-ordination, due to muscle weakness, muscle imbalance and joint stiffness.

Muscle weakness can be caused by inhibition of the muscles' controlling nerve systems due to pain or swelling in the knee, damage in the muscles, or simply lack of use. This reduces your ability to control the knee's movements and makes the knee unstable. Muscle imbalance involves relative weakness or tightness between muscle groups which should co-ordinate with each other.

All the muscles of the thigh begin to weaken and 'shrink' very quickly after any injury or in any painful condition. About an inch can be lost from the thigh girth within 12 to 24 hours of any injury. Inhibition of the vastus medialis obliquus happens virtually immediately once there is pain, swelling or damage in the knee. As control of the VMO is lost more quickly than control of the muscles with which it normally co-ordinates, an imbalance is set up. This imbalance is the inevitable result of knee pain or injury, and after any knee operation, and it has to be corrected if full functional recovery of the knee is to be achieved.

In some knee problems, the vastus medialis obliquus is undermined only to a very slight degree, for instance when there is only slight or intermittent pain. You may not be aware of the functional deficit, but even the slightest loss of VMO function is significant, as it represents a basic instability in the knee, and can lead to kneecap pain syndrome.

Joint imbalance means that interrelated joints are not functioning correctly, and can be part of a knee problem as cause or effect. You will probably find it harder to balance successfully standing on the injured leg, or to do leg movements which require fine control of the patterns of movement involving the foot, ankle, knee and hip.

Movement loss

Movement loss means you can no longer bend or straighten the knee fully, with or without your bodyweight on it. This can be a primary result of some internal obstruction or inflammation, or compensatory because of muscle tightness or habitual guarding of the knee.

Loss of mobility in the knee very often causes a reduction of movement in the ankle or hip on the same side. In some cases, a knee problem on one side leads to loss of movement in the other knee or hip, due to over-compensation or prolonged limping.

Movement loss can be due to muscle shortening. Tightness in the hamstring or gastrocnemius tendons is often the reason why you cannot straighten your knee fully. Quadriceps shortening, especially in the longest part of the muscle, rectus femoris, can prevent the knee from bending completely, especially when you lie on your stomach.

Changes in the joint surfaces, loose bodies inside the joint or damage to the knee's internal structures can block the knee's normal movements. If there is internal blockage, disease or severe degeneration, the knee tends to lose its ability to straighten out properly, and remains bent however hard you try to extend it. This is called fixed flexion deformity.

Kneecap pain syndrome

5

WHAT IS KNEECAP PAIN SYNDROME?

Kneecap pain syndrome is one of the most common problems to affect the knee. It causes a specific pain pattern related to the position and movement of the kneecap, and this is its main characteristic. It is commonly known by a variety of different names, including anterior knee pain (syndrome), patellar pain syndrome, retropatellar pain, patellar compression syndrome, patellar malalignment syndrome, patellalgia, patellar chondropathy, patellofemoral pain syndrome (PFPS), patellofemoral dysfunction, patellofemoral arthralgia, chondromalacia patellae, and 'runner's knee'.

It can occur as a primary condition, or secondary to another injury or pain syndrome in the knee. As a primary injury, kneecap pain can happen either through trauma or as a result of overuse. If pain in the kneecap is noticeable immediately after an injury to the front of the knee, it is primary and traumatic. The pain can be either severe or mild. Pain through overuse often comes on apparently without cause, although in fact there is always a reason for it. It can happen in either knee, dominant or non-dominant, in each knee in turn, or in both knees simultaneously. It can build up in a slow progression, or it can come on suddenly at an excruciatingly sharp level.

If the problem is secondary to some other knee condition, the pain may accompany the main injury, or it may develop gradually, either during the later stages of recovery from the main injury, or after the primary injury has been resolved. Whatever the cause of the kneecap pain syndrome, the pain and its intensity can fluctuate. The problem may be short-lived, or it can drag on, sometimes for several years.

What causes the pain?

It has been established that high compressive forces within the kneecap (patellofemoral) joint play an important part in kneecap pain syndrome. Faulty mechanics adversely affect the way the kneecap moves in relation to the thigh-bone. Painful pressure is created when the knee moves against the load of your bodyweight or a resistance.

In most cases, contrary to what you might expect, kneecap pain is not directly related to any notable damage to the kneecap or its related surface over the knuckle of the thigh-bone. Sometimes there is roughening, softening or pitting on the cartilage surface of the back of the kneecap, technically called chondromalacia patellae, which usually happens to younger patients as the result of trauma. In older age, there may be damage in the kneecap joint due to wear-and-tear degeneration (osteoarthritis). However, quite severe degrees of damage may be present on the kneecap joint surfaces without causing any knee pain. Conversely, there may be quite intense pain, yet little or even no sign of degeneration or injury in the articular cartilage. This is why it is inaccurate to use such terms as 'chondromalacia patellae' or 'retropatellar arthritis' as sole definitions for most or all cases of kneecap pain. It is more realistic to use generalized descriptive names, such as kneecap pain or patellofemoral pain syndrome.

It is unclear exactly how the nerve mechanisms give rise to the pain pattern typical of kneecap pain syndrome. What is clear in clinical practice is that the pain relates directly to the faulty mechanics which disrupt normal function in the kneecap joint. If the faulty mechanics are accurately corrected, the pain goes away, and will return only if there is another episode of injury or disturbance to the joint mechanics for any reason.

How does kneecap pain syndrome happen?

The most important feature of kneecap pain is reduced or lost function in the vastus medialis obliquus muscle just above the inner side of the knee, which is the only active controlling mechanism for the kneecap on that side. The muscle may become weak, inefficient or uncoordinated, and in extreme cases it stops functioning altogether.

The VMO is undermined immediately by direct trauma to the knee-cap. A fall on to the front of the knee or a knock, blow or kick to the kneecap will cause instant inhibition of the muscle, giving rise to primary front-knee pain. Any traumatic injury or pain syndrome affecting the knee joint as a whole also results in inhibition of the VMO, and this can give rise to kneecap pain alongside damage to some of the knee's structures. Kneecap pain is inevitable in any situation where the knee has been immobilized in the bent position for a length of time, for instance after certain types of leg fracture, or following some types of knee operation, such as surgery for the posterior cruciate ligament.

VMO deficiency and resultant kneecap pain can be related to an imbalance in the body's mechanics, so many different factors may be involved in the syndrome.

Growth, specifically bone development, can play a part. In the teens, anywhere between the ages of 13 and 16, there can be a marked growth spurt in the leg bones. In boys, this often causes shortening and therefore quite severe tightness in the hamstrings, which pull the knees from behind and prevent them from straightening out into the locked position, so blocking the VMO. In girls, the VMO can be undermined when the hips widen with the onset of puberty and alter the angle at which the quadriceps muscles exert their pull over the kneecap and knee joint.

Teenagers who have hyperextending knees (genu recurvatum) and high kneecaps (patella alta) tend to have inherently weak VMO muscles, and so are especially prone to developing primary kneecap pain. Knock-knee (genu valgum) or bow leg (genu varum) can also be a factor.

Malalignment of one or both hips or ankles can influence the onset of

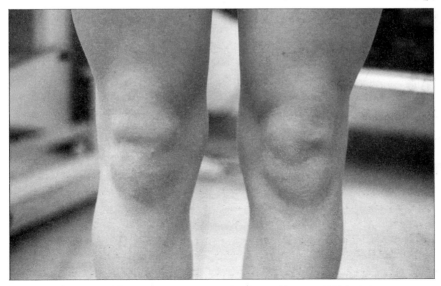

Vastus medialis obliquus deficiency of the right knee in a 10-year-old girl

kneecap pain. The Q-angle (which shows the alignment of the kneecap relative to the thigh-bone and shin-bone) may be larger or smaller than normal in cases of kneecap pain. The A-angle, which measures the position of the kneecap relative to the tibial tubercle, is likely to be larger than normal. Tightness in the iliotibial tract can pull the kneecap outwards and prevent its normal glide. Like shortened hamstrings, a tight iliotibial tract can also exert a negative influence on the VMO muscles. Faulty foot mechanics, especially over-pronation (inward twisting), can play a part in undermining the VMO and creating adverse pressure on the kneecap joint, both in the young and in adults.

Any previous knee injury which has not been fully and properly rehabilitated and has left a mechanical deficit can result in tightness at the back of the knee and VMO deficiency long after the original injury has apparently healed. A childhood or teenage knock on the knee can lead to kneecap pain, sometimes together with other knee problems, many years later. In the early teens, imperfect recovery from previous Osgood-Schlatter's syndrome (see p.81) predisposes to kneecap pain at any time within about two years. In older age, the knees can get drawn into the bent position by the effects of wear-and-tear degeneration (osteoarthritis), and this automatically reduces the efficiency of the VMO.

Muscle or tendon injuries anywhere in the thighs or lower legs can create a damaging imbalance affecting the kneecap joint mechanics, and perhaps the main knee joint, if full recovery of flexibility, strength and co-ordination is not achieved.

WHO GETS KNEECAP PAIN SYNDROME?

The kneecap pattern of pain can happen in one or both knees in males or females of any age, from earliest childhood to old age. It is particularly common among teenagers, especially females.

Any sport or activity which stresses the bent knee can give rise to the problem, so squash, fencing and kayaking, for instance, are risk sports in this regard. Runners are prone to kneecap pain, especially those athletes who train or race on hilly ground or on a camber, or who do excessive hopping and bounding exercises. Kneecap pain can happen to cyclists if the saddle is even marginally too low, and if they don't get out of the saddle to go up a slope or hill. Rowers may get it if the stretcher is too short or at the wrong angle to allow the legs to straighten out fully at the end of each stroke. Canoeists are vulnerable, because they balance in the boat by holding their legs slightly bent. Hill walking in heavy boots can easily set off the problem. Skiing in itself is less likely to cause kneecap pain than the popular pre-ski sit-squat exercise, where you perch against a wall with your knees bent at right angles in a sitting position (but without a chair) and stay there for as long as possible. There can be cumulative stress on the kneecap through repetitive bouncing on to the bent knee, as can happen in trampolining.

Failure to lock the knees straight after bending them can cause kneecap pain in weight-lifting, aerobics and many other activities. Doing knee extensions, whether using ankle weights, a weights boot or a knee extension machine, can be a direct cause of kneecap pain. If you do the exercise sitting on a horizontal surface you cannot lock the knees fully straight, so the vastus medialis obliquus is not activated properly in relation to the other front-thigh muscles. A common mistake when doing knee extensions is to work the front-thigh muscles only in their strongest middle range, rocking the knees backwards and forwards in the bent position, and neglecting the VMO. Instead you should place a support such as a rolled towel under your knees to lift them slightly in relation to your hips, make sure you lock your knees as straight as possible at the climax of the movement, then control the reverse motion so that you bend your knees slowly back to the starting position.

Kneecap pain is an occupational hazard for carpet-layers, electricians and gardeners, who have to kneel and crouch in their daily work. As it can also happen to people who have to sit still for long periods, students, office workers, cinema- and theatregoers, and those who simply 'sit around' all day are equally likely to get it. In one slightly unusual case, a teenage girl whom I was treating was not getting better as I had expected, until she confessed that her hobby of bell-ringing every week was hurting her knees. A short period of rest from bell-ringing while she worked at her treatment and rehabilitation exercises was then sufficient to solve the problem.

SIGNS AND SYMPTOMS OF KNEECAP PAIN SYNDROME

Typically, the pain feels fairly general, and patients often describe it as being 'around the whole knee', or over the whole front of the knee. Sometimes there is only one small painful area, somewhere close to the kneecap.

All the activities which bring on kneecap pain will remain painful until the problem is resolved. You may notice pain when the affected knee is bent under a load, as in squatting or crouching, kneeling, lifting weights from the floor, and going up and down stairs. The knee also tends to get painful and perhaps stiff if you sit still for long periods: this symptom is called the 'cinema sign', although it applies to any situation where you sit with the knee bent, whether working at a desk, watching television or on a long flight in an aeroplane. Sometimes sitting does not cause pain, but standing up from the sitting position gives a twinge. The knee may or may not hurt at night. If it does, it may ache as you lie still, or twinge if you move or turn over awkwardly. The knee will hurt more if any direct pressure is exerted on it, for example wearing tight trousers or a constricting bandage.

The knee may seem to give way when it is bent under a load, perhaps as you step down from a kerb, but it rarely gives way to the extent that you fall over. You may notice a slight swelling or puffiness around the front of the knee, and in some cases the knee may feel warm or hot.

HOW KNEECAP PAIN SYNDROME IS DIAGNOSED

The practitioner treating you has to take care to differentiate kneecap pain syndrome from the other conditions which can cause a similar pain pattern. In particular, he or she will exclude bipartite or tripartite patella, kneecap subluxation, stress fracture of the kneecap, bursitis, tendinitis, osteochondritis and pain referred from the hip. As in all cases of knee pain, the practitioner will also be aware of the possibility of more serious causes, such as inflammation, infection or disease.

Your description of the pain pattern is crucial, and you must describe every situation in which you feel pain, and any in which there is no pain.

When the practitioner examines you, he or she will expect to find that the vastus medialis obliquus muscle is not functioning efficiently and is weak, and that the kneecap is not tracking correctly in its groove. The front-thigh muscles are likely to be tight. The back of the knee may be tender on pressure. There may be slight swelling in the front of the knee around the edges of the kneecap.

Tests for vastus medialis obliquus insufficiency

If the vastus medialis obliquus muscle is not functioning efficiently, you may have difficulty tightening the thigh muscles with your leg straight to make the kneecap twitch, and it may be even harder for you to release the muscles once they have contracted. This test is more difficult when you are standing up than when you are sitting on the couch. If the VMO is weak, you will find it hard to lock your knee straight to its fullest extent. When you are sitting on the couch with your leg straight, you will not be able to lock the knee into full extension and maintain the position. If only

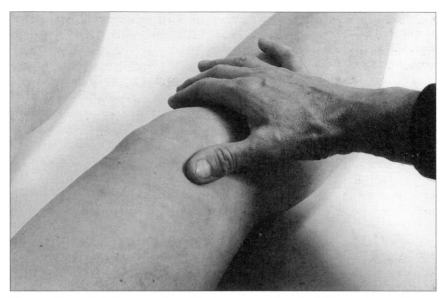

The practitioner feels the outer side of the kneecap as the patient tightens the quadriceps muscles to test for patellar deviation

one knee is affected, there will be a noticeable difference between the performance of the VMO muscles in each leg. If you try to straighten both knees fully, lifting your heels off the supporting surface, the heel on the side of the weakened VMO will not be lifted as high as the other foot.

Tests for patellar tracking

If your kneecap is not tracking correctly, it will deviate noticeably instead of gliding straight up and down in the line of the thigh when you tighten the quadriceps muscles to straighten the knee (although a slight deviation is considered normal in a painless knee). For this test, you sit on the couch with your legs straight in the neutral position first. If your knee is not too sensitive, you may be asked to sit on the side of the couch and straighten your knee from the bent position.

In almost all cases, the deviation of the kneecap is towards the outer (lateral) side of the knee and thigh, under the overriding influence of the strong central and outer parts of the quadriceps muscle group, and of the iliotibial band. The kneecap may also be out of true when it is at rest in its groove, with the knee straight and relaxed. Very often it is pulled over and downwards towards the outer side, so that instead of the bone being more or less horizontal, its outer border is tethered down and its inner border is tilted upwards. Measuring the Q- and A-angles can give an idea of the position of the kneecap, but there is considerable doubt whether these measurements are accurate and reliable enough to be of real significance when assessing knee problems.

To check the back of your knee, the practitioner will ask you to lie face down, so that he or she can feel the tissues by hand. Gentle pressure will establish whether the tendons at the back of the knee are tight or tender. The flexibility of your front-thigh muscles is checked while you are in the same position. The practitioner will ask you to bend your knees actively, one at a time. Then you will relax your legs, and the practitioner will gently bend your knees passively.

X-rays and investigations

For an objective image of the position of the kneecaps, special X-rays called skyline or Merchant views can be taken to show the position and tilt of the kneecaps as they rest across the thigh-bones when the joints are fully bent. For more detailed information about the state of the kneecap joint, if there is doubt about the diagnosis, the doctor or surgeon may request an MRI scan, computerized tomography, an isotope scan, or a double contrast arthrograph. Blood tests may be taken if there is any chance that the knee pain is associated with inflammation, illness or some kind of joint disease.

Tests for kneecap sensitivity

There are three specific tests for establishing whether the kneecap is especially sensitive, and these will always cause pain if you have kneecap pain syndrome. First, when you are sitting on the couch with your legs straight and supported, the practitioner will glide the kneecap sideways in each direction to feel whether there is localized tenderness when the underside of the bone is rubbed with a finger. Second, the practitioner will press down on the kneecap to grind it against the adjacent surface of the thigh-bone. Third, the practitioner will place his or her hand on your thigh, resting the web between the thumb and index finger against the upper edge of your kneecap, and will ask you to tense your thigh muscles to straighten your knee while he or she blocks the kneecap's movement upwards along the thigh. This test is called 'Clarke's sign'.

Personally, I never do any of these tests, as the first does not necessarily prove where the patient's pain originates, and the other two inevitably cause quite a high level of pain, further inhibiting the VMO, and in many cases undermining the patient's confidence in the practitioner. If there is clear evidence of functional pain relating to the kneecap joint, obvious insufficiency in the vastus medialis obliquus, and no sign of any other type of injury or condition, that is sufficient to justify treating the problem as front-knee pain.

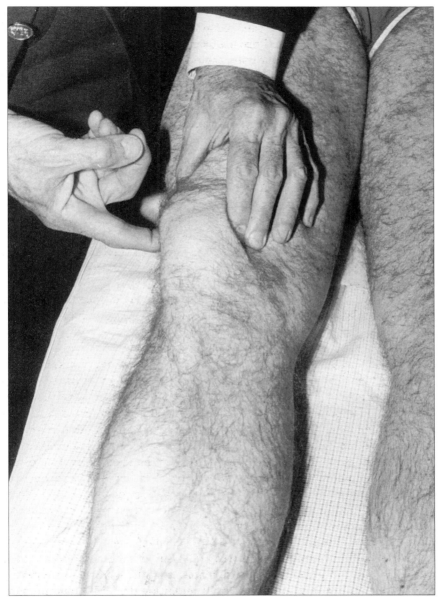

Testing the underside of the kneecap for tenderness

TREATMENT FOR KNEECAP PAIN SYNDROME

It is generally accepted that the majority of kneecap pain cases are best treated conservatively, usually by a physiotherapist using rehabilitation exercises, rather than with surgery.

VMO revival: the primary concern of treatment

In my practice, I focus on reviving correct and accurate function in the vastus medialis obliquus as the essential prerequisite for getting rid of front-knee pain in order to return to full physical activities.

The patient has to understand how the VMO should work, and be aware that the VMO is not working properly in order to work on the fine control of the muscle, which is the necessary basis for its correct activity. I always use electrical neuromuscular stimulation to help the patient regain co-ordination of the VMO (see p.147). Throughout the patient's workout with the muscle stimulator, I mobilize the kneecap towards the inner side of the knee between contractions, partly to correct any lateral tilting, partly to check that the muscles have relaxed completely.

In long-standing (chronic) cases, the patient may find it difficult, even impossible, to contract the VMO at all, never mind regaining control of the muscle's finer function. In this case, the patient usually benefits from investing in a small muscle stimulator. Using the stimulator regularly and

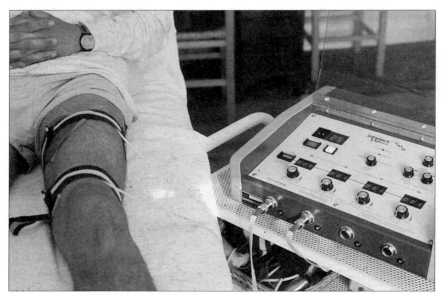

Electrical muscle stimulation for the VMO

frequently at home helps to counteract the harmful effects of the numerous positions and movements in daily life which would otherwise undermine the VMO.

The home stimulator is also an investment for the future, because it means that the patient can immediately re-start self-treatment if the knee starts to ache or hurt again. If there is a recurrence of kneecap pain, early use of the muscle stimulator might prevent it from developing into a real problem, although of course you should refer back to your practitioner quickly if the problem does not respond. Use of the muscle stimulator as a self-help treatment is perfectly safe, provided that you follow the instructions and guidelines given by your physiotherapist with due care.

Treatment for related factors

While regaining VMO efficiency is my top priority, I also take into account any subsidiary factors relating to the front-knee pain syndrome. If the structures at the back of the knee are tense and tight, I release them using massage or gentle soft-tissue manipulation. If there is tightness in the soft tissues attached to the upper outer edge of the kneecap, I release them with soft-tissue manipulation. If the iliotibial band is particularly tight, I release it manually and with guided stretching techniques. When knee-bending in the front-lying position is limited, I do assisted stretching techniques for the front-thigh muscles, and, if necessary, gentle

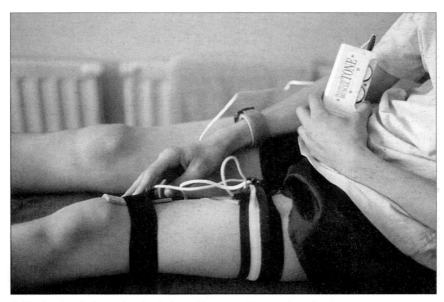

Self-help electrical muscle stimulation with a portable stimulator for home use

manipulation to free the knee's rotatory movements. If the patient has hyperextending knees and lax hamstrings, I introduce the exercises to make the hamstrings firmer. For stiffness in the hip, I mobilize the joint with manual therapy. If the foot mechanics are faulty, I use guided movements to help correct them. When there are very marked problems in the foot, and they are definitely playing a part in the patient's pain cycle, I recommend the patient to a podiatrist in case orthotics might help (see p.113)

In some cases, food intolerance (see p.46) and stress (p.41) complicate the condition and have to be addressed.

Self-help for Kneecap Pain Syndrome

The core of the patient's self-help programme is the exercise regime designed to regain VMO efficiency and co-ordination (see pp.158–64, exercises 1–11). The exercises should be done meticulously at least twice a day. Knee-straightening movements should be incorporated into your everyday life, if this is at all possible.

If it helps, you can use a simple patellar strap made out of a tubular bandage to relieve the pressure on the kneecap. The strap is placed just

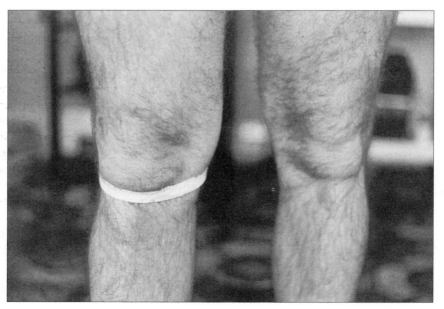

The patellar strap

under the lower tip of the kneecap, so that it passes round the soft pads at the front of the knee. It should not feel tight. It may reduce your discomfort when going up or down stairs, and you may find it helpful to wear it when you have to walk around. You should remove the strap if it no longer seems to help or if it gets uncomfortable.

In the first phase of recovery, while the knee is still painful to bend under a load, you must, as far as possible, avoid stressing the bent knee. Avoid sitting still or kneeling for long periods: get up, stretch and walk around whenever possible. While sitting, try to sit on the edge of your chair at intervals, so that you can place your heel on the floor and practise straightening your knee. On no account should you squat, or sit with your legs twisted and tucked underneath you. Adjust your car seat, so that your legs can stretch out as straight as possible. You should avoid stairs, but if you must, you may find it easier to climb stairs if you go up on your toes as soon as your foot is placed on the step. Going down stairs may be less painful if you come down with your body turned slightly sideways.

Any activity which causes pain must be avoided, although you can safely continue any sports or hobbies which are painless. You may or may not, for instance, be able to ride a bicycle without pain if the saddle is high enough to allow the knee to straighten out, and if you get out of the saddle when going up slopes.

PROGRESSING THE REHABILITATION PROGRAMME

As soon as VMO function has improved, and the symptoms have abated – so that, for instance, you no longer notice pain on stairs or when sitting still – you may progress to active exercises which bend the knee under load. Running may be possible, especially if you run fast rather than jog slowly, and if you include some spells of running backwards within a running session. Running backwards has been shown to reduce the compressive forces on the kneecap joint to a significant degree. Quick half-squats standing up are progressed to slow knee-bending movements, and ultimately to full knee-bends.

Even after you have made a full recovery, you should maintain the protective knee-straightening exercises indefinitely, or at least for several weeks after you have re-started your normal activities.

HOW LONG TO FULL RECOVERY?

In some cases, one session of treatment including VMO muscle stimulation for twenty to thirty minutes can be sufficient to restore efficient neuromuscular co-ordination in the VMO, and therefore to cure the kneecap pain. In this case, you should still do the rehabilitation exercise programme for at least six weeks, but you can safely resume normal activities and sports during this period, providing that each new activity is introduced gradually. More often, recovery extends over a space of weeks. It all depends on how long it takes you to regain full control over the VMO muscle.

In long-standing (chronic) cases, recovery can take several months, but so long as the diagnosis is correct, and no new complicating factors intervene, it is always possible to effect a cure for the symptoms, in my experience. This confidence helps the patient to be motivated to persevere with the programme until recovery is reached.

When an extended treatment programme is necessary, I usually treat patients with kneecap pain once or twice a week to begin with, spacing out the treatments to monitor progress over a period of time until full recovery is achieved.

OTHER TREATMENT METHODS FOR KNEECAP PAIN SYNDROME

Other practitioners, of course, may treat front-knee pain syndrome using different methods. Many have a good success rate, although there is still a widespread belief that the condition is difficult to treat, so presumably some practitioners are not confident of solving the problem.

Some practitioners use electrical muscle stimulation for the VMO, but with the knee bent rather than straight. Others use biofeedback rather than muscle stimulation to re-train the VMO's controlling nerve to fire properly. One of the most widely used and accepted systems for treating kneecap pain is the McConnell technique, devised by the Australian physiotherapist Jenny McConnell, which provides a re-training schedule for the kneecap joint's controlling muscles, in conjunction with a precise method of taping the kneecap in order to limit its pain-causing movements.

Surgery is definitely the very last resort for kneecap pain syndrome. Removing the kneecap (patellectomy) is a drastic solution which in fact has very poor results, not least because the recovery of reasonable knee function is extremely difficult. It is rarely used now as a cure for kneecap

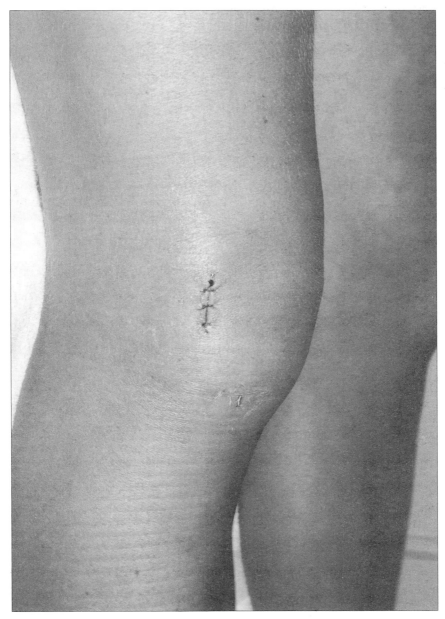

The scar from the lateral release operation

pain. More often, when all else has failed, the surgical procedure chosen is the lateral release, which simply cuts through the tight tissues binding the kneecap down towards the outer side of the knee, in order to allow the bone free gliding movement in the right track. This operation can produce good results, although the knee may be quite painful during the first few days post-operatively, and recovery can be relatively slow. When the lateral release fails to provide a cure, it is most often because the rehabilitation programme focusing on the VMO has not been carried out, so that the knee's functional and protective mechanisms have not been regained.

KNEECAP PAIN: RECOVERY AND RECURRENCE

The problem is over once you can sit still, go up and down stairs, and squat down freely without pain.

Kneecap pain is likely to recur if you ever neglect the vastus medialis obliquus muscle, either through careless posture, or through doing activities which overwork the other front-thigh muscles to the detriment of their balance with the VMO. If you have had kneecap pain previously, you are more likely to get it again as a secondary effect if you hurt any other part of your knee.

If the problem does come back, you should immediately start doing the basic protective and remedial programme for the VMO. If you have your own small muscle stimulator, you should try using it to revive the VMO. If self-help measures do not solve the problem within a few days, refer back to your practitioner for assessment and further treatment. This is also a safeguard, in case the pain is not really a recurrence of kneecap pain syndrome, but due to some other problem.

Bone injuries and problems

6

TRAUMATIC FRACTURES OF THE BONES

A severe external force can cause a bone break in the thigh-bone, shin-bone or kneecap. Fractures are categorized according to the amount and type of damage involved. When a bone breaks without causing any surface damage to the skin, the fracture is called simple. Where the skin is broken, the fracture is open, and if the broken bone is visible through the wound, it is a compound fracture. When other internal structures such as blood vessels and nerves are involved in the bone injury, it is a complicated fracture. A shattered bone is called a comminuted fracture. When a bone is crushed into itself, the fracture is impacted or compressed. If part of a bone is broken off because the tendon or ligament attached to it has held firm under stress, it is an avulsion fracture. Damage to the articular cartilage in conjunction with the bone break is termed an osteochondral fracture. Children's fractures of long bones like the shin-bone are called greenstick fractures, because the resilient immature bone tends to bend and crack rather than break right through.

Fractures in the thigh-bone and shin-bone

In the adult, the thigh-bone and shin-bone are extremely strong. They are reasonably well protected by the ligaments and other soft tissues which bind them together. A severe disruptive force will damage the soft tissues without necessarily causing bone damage. It takes a very violent force to damage the bones, and in many cases the bone damage is accompanied by injury to the soft tissues.

The accident may involve a direct blow, for instance through an awkward fall from a ladder, a bad tackle in football (soccer), or a collision with another skier at speed; it might be a crush injury, as can happen in a motorbike accident or when a horse falls on to its rider; there may be compression, for instance through a bad landing from a parachute jump; or shearing forces can be involved, as when a skier falls with a foot trapped in an unreleased boot binding. Very often the bone fracture is caused by a combination of forces.

In children and teenagers, the knee bones are much more vulnerable to damage through adverse forces, because the growth plates are relatively weak until their fusion processes are complete. The type of accident which would perhaps cause medial or lateral ligament damage in the adult is more likely to cause a physeal (growth plate) fracture in the young patient. For this reason, it should never be assumed that any significant traumatic injury in a young person is simply ligament damage until the bones have been checked, which may be done by X-ray or scanning.

Kneecap, tibial tubercle and fibular fractures

Being a free-floating bone which does not bear the body's weight, the kneecap is less vulnerable to traumatic fracture. It can be broken through a direct fall from a height on to the kneecap. Indirect pressure exerted through the quadriceps muscles, especially when the knee is fully bent, can split the kneecap or cause avulsion fractures at the edges of the kneecap or the tibial tubercle, for instance when a footballer is blocked while contracting the quadriceps muscles hard just before kicking the ball. Avulsion fractures are especially likely to happen in teenagers during their vulnerable growth periods.

The fibula (outer leg-bone) is not a weightbearing bone. It is much less strong than the shin-bone, and can be broken together with the shin-bone in a major accident, or on its own through a more minor force which hits the bone directly. If it is broken near the head of the bone just under the knee, the lateral popliteal nerve which winds round this part of the bone may be damaged, causing peculiar sensations of tingling or numbness down the leg into the foot, or a kind of partial paralysis called 'foot-drop' (see p.77).

Possible treatments for traumatic fractures

Any fracture involving the bones is of course treated as an emergency, because of the outpouring of blood which inevitably accompanies it. Fractured bones are treated according to the type of fracture, severity of injury and sometimes the age of the patient. The decision is taken by the orthopaedic surgeon. When possible, the patient is offered a choice of alternative treatments, with an explanation of what each entails.

In some cases the damaged bone is simply protected in a plaster cast.

The patient is soon allowed to move about on crutches, usually avoiding taking weight through the leg at first, and then gradually putting more weight through the foot after a weightbearing rocker has been added to the plaster. The patient has to be especially careful to look after the circulatory flow in the leg (see p.177) and must refer to the consultant or general practitioner if there is any sign of congestion, interruption to the normal blood flow or burning sensations.

Very often, the surgeon operates to fix the broken bone with a metal plate, pin or screws. The fixation is usually internal, inserted into the bone under the skin, but it can be external, so that it looks like a kind of cage round the bone. The external fixation is removed as soon as the bone heals adequately. Internal fixation may be left in indefinitely or removed after a space of time, which might be a year after the operation. Sometimes the decision to remove the internal fixator is made because the metal has started to cause a kind of irritation, a feeling that it is 'in the way', even though there is no infection or urgent reason for removing it.

If at all possible, knee movement is preserved and encouraged. If the patient has a period of bed-rest in hospital, knee movement is often kept going by a machine called Continuous Passive Motion (CPM) which bends and straightens the joint gently. This can be left on for hours at a time, and ensures that there is a good flow of blood through the knee and the whole leg, even though the patient is lying still. Maintenance exercises which preserve muscle tone and circulatory flow without stressing the fractured bone are usually strongly encouraged from the earliest stage of recovery.

During the healing period, the surgeon monitors the bone healing, usually by taking X-rays at intervals. This dictates when weightbearing through the leg is started. Weightbearing has to be progressive, as dictated by the surgeon and controlled by the physiotherapist. The specialist paediatric surgeon will monitor a child's broken bone extra-carefully during the healing period. If the growth area (physis) was involved in the fracture, there is sometimes a risk that the bone's growth will be disrupted, so that the bone grows too large or fails to develop properly.

Recovery from any major fracture of the leg-bones takes several months. Healing starts virtually immediately after the fracture, but the shin-bone and thigh-bone take about three months to regain basic strength, and another three months to consolidate. The bones can take up to a year to strengthen up to their previous level after a fracture, so there is a risk of re-fracture if any unexpected excessive pressure is applied to the bone while it is still vulnerable. The fibula heals more quickly than the shin-bone, and can recover functionally within three to six months, depending on the type and severity of the fracture. Bone healing can be slowed down if there has been an infection or circulatory problem, or if the patient's diet is inadequate. Failure to knit together again is called non-union. A specific type of electrical stimulation can sometimes help the bone to mend, but surgical treatment to activate the bone healing process is often required.

KNEE DISLOCATION

Dislocation is a distortion of a joint which does not correct itself spontaneously. This differentiates it from subluxation, where the joint comes apart but goes back into place immediately.

Dislocation of the tibiofemoral joint is a major traumatic injury, which must always be treated as an emergency. When the knee dislocates, the bones separate from each other and their binding tissues. As it takes a very violent force, several of the soft tissues are usually torn as the knee gives way, and there are often fractures in the shin-bone or thigh-bone as well. The dislocation can happen in any direction: the shin-bone can be pulled forwards or backwards relative to the thigh-bone if the cruciate ligaments or joint capsule are torn; there can be a sideways dislocation when the medial or lateral ligaments give way; or the thigh-bone and shin-bone can be twisted on each other if most of the soft tissues are torn together.

The type of accident in which knee dislocation happens usually involves heavy pressure against the leg, as in a bad fall when skiing, an awkward landing from a parachute jump, a tackle in which an opponent falls across the player's outstretched leg in soccer, American football or rugby, or when a horse falls and traps its rider's leg in show-jumping or hunting.

An experienced qualified doctor or surgeon may manipulate the knee back into position at the moment of the accident. This should never be attempted by non-professional first-aiders, as there is a risk of causing serious damage to the knee's major blood vessels and nerves. The injury itself can cause rupture of one of the leg's main arteries, so the casualty must be taken to hospital as quickly as possible. If the bleeding is not stopped, gangrene could develop, although this is mercifully rare.

Surgery is usually needed to repair the torn tissues. Afterwards, the leg may be protected in a plaster cast, and progressive exercises started carefully under the guidance of a physiotherapist. Throughout the recovery period, the patient must take care of the circulation in the leg and refer to the doctor or surgeon urgently if there are any danger signs, like a burning sensation or a feeling of cramp or constriction.

One complication of knee dislocation can be damage to the nerve which winds round the head of the fibula close to the knee, the lateral popliteal branch of the common peroneal nerve. This causes a type of paralysis called 'foot-drop', which prevents the patient from lifting the foot up at the ankle. The problem may not be obvious at first. If it shows up at a later stage, nerve conduction tests may be needed to confirm the nerve damage. Treatment may be needed, and the knee usually recovers with time, but nerve damage can extend the recovery period by several weeks.

Overall recovery from knee dislocation takes many months. The joint movement may remain permanently slightly limited, but knee function is usually good enough for most normal activities including non-contact sports.

KNEECAP DISLOCATION AND SUBLUXATION

If the kneecap is displaced, it is almost always outwards, although it can go inwards in the rare event of the lateral structures and binding tissues giving way. Kneecap subluxation or dislocation happens most commonly in situations when the knee is bent under load and the inner muscles, especially vastus medialis obliquus, cannot hold the kneecap in place. The force needed to cause displacement of the kneecap is not necessarily great,

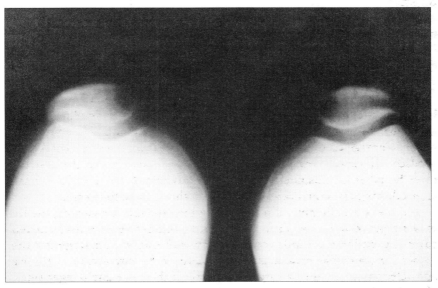

Skyline X-rays showing subluxation of the kneecap on the left side of the picture

if the muscles around the kneecap are weakened or unbalanced. The background factors which can contribute to these injuries are similar to those influencing kneecap pain syndrome (see pp.57–72). Kneecap displacement is especially common among female teenagers, although it can happen to males, young children and adults as well.

Both subluxation and dislocation tend to be recurring injuries after the first episode, and both can result in kneecap pain syndrome. The pain may be imprecise, but the displacement causes a feeling of something going out of place. The knee may feel as though it will give way when this happens. If the kneecap joint is very unstable, surgery may be needed. There are various possible operations to stabilize the kneecap. The simplest is the lateral release operation, through which the lateral structures are loosened to allow the kneecap more freedom. More complicated procedures can involve reconstruction of the tissues on the front of the knee, to alter the alignment between the kneecap and the patellar tendon.

Whether or not the problem is treated surgically, it is vital in all cases to regain full function in vastus medialis obliquus together with its proper co-ordination with the other knee muscles.

STRESS FRACTURES AND OVERUSE BONE INJURIES

A stress fracture is an overuse syndrome in which a bone cracks due to cumulative repetitive pressure on a particular part of the bone. This type of fracture can happen in any bone in the body, including the bones around the knee. The cause of the stress fracture is less to do with jarring than with pressure caused by the tension of a muscle or tendon pulling against the bone. In growing children, the bones are vulnerable to overuse stresses which can prevent them from knitting together in the normal way. This type of injury is very similar to a stress fracture.

Causes of stress fractures

The primary cause of the stress fracture is over-activity in relation to the strength of the bone. The stress fracture is usually associated with repetitive sports such as long-distance running, but any activity carried out repetitively can cause similar bone damage, for instance drill practices where a single technique or pattern of movement is done over and over again for sports like soccer, tennis, squash or hockey, which normally involve varied movements. Normally the cause of the stress fracture is a sudden increase of repetitive activity which the bones cannot cope with.

This may be an increase in mileage for marathon training or winter endurance work for track runners, or resuming training after a break for sickness or holidays. New recruits for the armed services are particularly vulnerable if they are not properly prepared for training exercises involving forced marches over difficult terrain carrying heavy loads. Doing repetitive training on consecutive days, without allowing for recovery in between sessions, is extremely likely to lead to stress fractures.

Stress fractures can happen at any age to males and females alike, although they are more likely to happen if you have some dietary deficiency which has affected the mineral content of your bones. In female long-distance runners there may be a link between being very thin, lack of menstruation (amenorrhoea) and stress fractures. Background factors to the stress fracture can include muscle tightness, muscle imbalance, circulatory inefficiency including varicose veins, and faulty joint mechanics affecting the foot, ankle, knee or hip.

Around the knee, the stress fracture can happen in the shin-bone or thigh-bone through running, repetitive kicking or aerobics class exercises. It can also happen in the kneecap as a result of sports which involve repetitive forceful bending of the knee, like squash, cycling hard with the saddle too low, or running or walking up and down hills for long distances or days on end. In children, if the kneecap fails to fuse properly, it is called a bipartite or tripartite patella according to how many parts there are, and this can cause pain similar to that of a stress fracture. The same activities can also cause excessive pressure and therefore stress fracture in the tibial tubercle at the top of the shin-bone through the pull of the patellar tendon which is attached to it.

The pain pattern of stress fractures

At first there is only slight pain *after* the activity which is causing the problem. There may be a dull ache at night. The pain increases if the activity is continued, and it begins to be felt during the repetitive activity. With a few days' rest, the pain subsides very quickly, but it recurs immediately if training is resumed. In a very few cases, the pain develops to a severe degree and the bone breaks right through, which puts a stop to repetitive training. More often, the pain remains at a low level, warning that the problem is still there without actually preventing the activities which stress the area. The pattern of reduction and aggravation of pain in relation to activities and rest can continue almost indefinitely. Sports which do not involve repetitive movements, meanwhile, can usually be continued without causing any problems.

How stress fractures are identified

The first clue to the presence of a stress fracture is the history of how the pain started in relation to your activities. The bone is usually tender on direct pressure when the practitioner palpates it. The skin over the area may feel slightly warm, and sometimes looks slightly reddened. X-rays do not show the stress fracture until it is healing, so they are not useful for diagnosis. A clear X-ray may mislead you into thinking that the bone cannot be damaged, when in fact it can mean that the bone is cracked and has not started healing yet. A bone scan shows the damaged area as a 'hot spot', and this confirms the stress fracture in conjunction with the typical pain pattern. In most cases, the bone scan, which is an expensive procedure, is not necessary. However, if there is any doubt about the diagnosis, the specialist will probably order further investigations such as blood tests as well as the bone scan, to exclude the possibility of disease or bone tumour.

How stress fractures are treated

Once the stress fracture has been diagnosed, or established as the likely cause of your pain, you must rest for several weeks from any painful activities, and especially the activity which caused the problem. If you give in to the temptation to 'try out' the leg when it seems to feel better after a couple of weeks, you will simply prolong the injury. During the recovery period you should do exercise of any kind which is painless. Swimming and pool exercises are usually safe, and you may be able to run in shallow water, preferably varying direction to run not only forwards but backwards and sideways. You may even be able to do sports which involve varied weightbearing movements like badminton or squash if your injury was not associated with these.

Alternative training is an important part of promoting healing of the damaged bone. Complete rest can hinder the healing process, so it is not usual to immobilize the bone in a plaster cast, unless there is some particular reason for doing so. If there is pain on walking, the patient may be given crutches to reduce the amount of weight transmitted through the damaged bone. Some patients may be fitted with a removable cast to prevent accidental knocks against the bone. Pool work and non-weightbearing floor exercises have to be done as often as possible to help the bone to heal.

It is also important to stimulate the circulation, to help the healing. If there are background factors such as dietary deficiencies or poor foot mechanics, these are usually addressed with the help of the dietician, podiatrist or other appropriate specialist.

The normal period of relative rest is a minimum of eight weeks, although in certain cases it can be longer. Your specialist may repeat the bone scan to make sure that the stress fracture has healed, but usually the evidence of a long period without pain coupled with a reduction in tenderness is sufficient to allow a gradual return to normal activities.

The vital part of avoiding recurrence of the stress fracture, or a stress fracture in some other bone, is to space out any exercise sessions involving repetitive movements. I recommend the patient to start with one session a week for the first month, two in the second, and three in the third. The sessions are increased only if there is no hint of pain as a result of the activity. I prefer athletes not to do repetitive training, especially distance running, more than four times a week at the most. If they really feel they have to train five days a week or more, they must be warned to step up to running on consecutive days with great caution, and to rest from running if there is any sign of pain or muscle stiffness which does not ease quickly with careful stretching.

How to prevent stress fractures

Prevention of this overuse syndrome is best achieved by varying training and doing background fitness and conditioning work for good body balance. Training and practice routines specific to a sport should always be combined with protective exercise. Repetitive training on consecutive days should be avoided, and interspersed with different kinds of physical activity.

OSGOOD-SCHLATTER'S CONDITION

In children during the early teenage years, the bony attachment where the patellar tendon joins the tibial tubercle can become irritated and disrupted by excessive pressure from the tendon. This is an overuse syndrome which happens when the tibial tubercle is going through the fusion process of fixing itself on to the shin-bone. It usually happens somewhere between the ages of 12 and 16, and there may be a visible generalized growth spurt at the same time. The cause, symptoms and effects are very similar to those of a stress fracture in the same bone in an adult, but it is a much more common problem in youngsters because of the growth process of bone fusion. It is technically an apophysitis, and has a special name, Osgood-Schlatter's 'disease', although it is not a disease but a mechanical problem caused by excessive activity in relation to the bone's strength at the time.

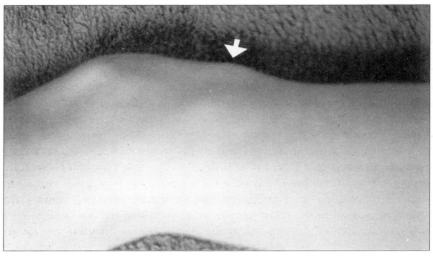

The visible deformity (arrowed) of Osgood-Schlatter's condition

How Osgood-Schlatter's condition happens

Osgood-Schlatter's condition is especially common among young soccer players, squash players and athletes. It can happen simply because of growth, when the youngster is doing his or her normal level of activities. It can be triggered by a change of routine, such as more intensive training and match-playing when the season starts.

The pain can start gradually or suddenly, and can range from a mild ache to sharp or severe pain. It is specifically located over the tibial tubercle, sometimes to one side of the bone or the other. The bone is tender on direct pressure and the area may feel warm to the touch. There may also be some swelling around the bone, and the bone itself can look abnormally prominent. The pain is felt during any movements which stress the knee in the bent position, so running, jumping, hopping, kicking and kneeling are all painful. Rest eases the pain, but it starts up again very quickly when stressful activities are undertaken. If the problem is allowed to develop to a severe stage, the knee muscles become weak, especially vastus medialis obliquus, and the joint may be fixed in the slightly bent position. In the worst of cases, the tibial tubercle becomes so frail that it gives way under pressure in an avulsion fracture.

How to cure Osgood-Schlatter's condition

The cure for Osgood-Schlatter's condition depends on rest from any painful activities. Ice applications and gentle massage round the painful area, perhaps with arnica or a heparinoid cream, can help to relieve the pain and stimulate the circulation. Any secondary problems, such as stiffness in the hip or poor foot mechanics, should be treated.

A programme of remedial exercises to restore and improve muscle function around the knee must be followed. The quadriceps and the hamstring muscles have to be stretched carefully and frequently, to prevent movement limitation. If the vastus medialis muscle is especially weakened, electrical muscle stimulation should be used to revive it (see p.147). Physical exercise helps to stimulate the circulation and promote healing, so the patient is encouraged to do any sports which do not cause pain. Swimming and cycling are usually good forms of painless alternative exercise. Putting the knee in a plaster cast makes it harder to engage in alternative physical activities, but this is sometimes done simply to prevent the patient from running around if persuasion has not worked.

Osgood-Schlatter's condition usually takes several weeks to clear up. It takes time for the remedial exercise programme to have its effect, and time must also be allowed for the growth spurt to be completed. The patient should not be allowed to return to the sports which caused pain until he or she can squat down comfortably and straighten the knee fully without pain. If sports are resumed too early, before the problem is properly resolved, the pain can persist for a year or even two, and, worse still, can lead to permanent limitation of movement in the affected knee which may cause more problems in later life.

OSTEOARTHRITIS AND DEGENERATIVE ARTHRITIS

Osteoarthritis is a condition in which the articular cartilage surfaces within a joint are damaged, usually through inflammation. A tendency to osteoarthritis can be hereditary, and it can affect virtually any joint in the body. The fingers, thumbs, elbows, hips and knees tend to be especially vulnerable. Osteoarthritis can cause episodes of acute pain and inflammation in which the affected joint(s) become very tender, sore, reddened, and often hot. It can also be present without causing any symptoms at all, even when very marked degenerative changes are visible on X-ray. A degree of osteoarthritis is likely to affect the majority of people over the age of 60, but people who have inherited the vulnerability to it can suffer from early adulthood.

Injuries or infections in a joint can set up a cycle of chronic swelling, leading to inflammation and therefore degeneration in the joint surfaces. This process can cause degeneration years after a significant injury to the

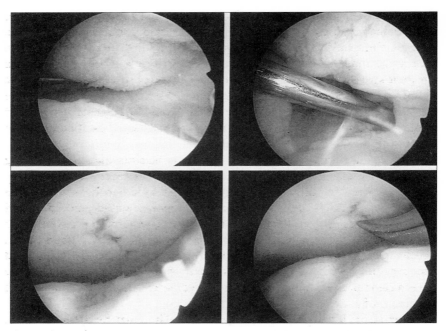

Damage to the articular cartilage in a patient with medial semilunar cartilage injury, seen at arthroscopy

affected joint. The degenerative changes are very similar to those of hereditary osteoarthritis, so the terms osteoarthritis and degenerative arthritis are often used interchangeably, but some specialists prefer to distinguish between degenerative arthritis resulting from previous injury and osteoarthritis arising as part of a hereditary condition. In some cases, of course, both types of degenerative change can be present together.

Knee injuries are especially likely to lead to later degenerative changes if the trauma caused bleeding into the joint and it was not removed quickly; if the injury was not diagnosed and treated efficiently, so that it led to repeated episodes of locking or giving way; or if recovery was incomplete and left mechanical imbalance and functional deficits. Degenerative changes in the knees are more likely to cause problems if the patient is overweight or has circulatory problems such as varicose veins. Excessive development of the front-thigh muscles relative to the hamstrings, as can happen through powerlifting, can give rise to damaging compressive forces on the knees which contribute to painful degenerative changes. Food intolerance (see p.46) can also play a part.

When degenerative changes in the knee are well advanced, there may be visible deformity and an obvious loss of joint mobility. The knee may be drawn inwards (genu valgum) or outwards (genu varum), depending on whether the inner or outer compartment of the joint is affected. The knee is almost always held in the bent position, or flexion deformity. On X-ray the shape of the joint surfaces looks abnormal. There may be loss of joint space, so that the bones are close together or even touching. The rounded condyles may become flattened. Jutting projections of bone called osteophytes may appear in the joint. Sometimes particles break off from the joint surface leaving erosions and forming loose bodies in the joint.

Appropriate exercise is vital for improving the situation and preventing degenerative changes from getting progressively worse. Excessive load-bearing, as in long-distance running or walking, has to be avoided. The right combination is moderate walking or running within pain limits and using shock-absorbing insoles, other types of general exercise such as swimming or cycling, and protective exercises to maintain good vastus medialis function and joint mobility (see pp.157–70). Immobility should be avoided, such as sitting or standing still for long periods. The overweight patient should follow a reducing diet, preferably under the guidance of a dietician.

Treatments aiming to control pain and swelling may be needed. A wide range of modalities can help, including anti-inflammatory drugs from the doctor, homoeopathic remedies, physiotherapy treatments, acupuncture, reflexology or healing. However, if the degeneration causes severely disabling pain and stiffness in the knee, replacing the joint with an artificial one may become the best option. Following the total knee replacement operation, effective rehabilitation is vital if the patient is to make the best possible recovery. It should be possible to return to moderate sporting activities including walking and golf after the operation, but the type and amount of exercise allowed must be dictated by the surgeon.

OSTEOCHONDRITIS DISSECANS

In teenagers, and sometimes in younger children, a certain kind of damage can happen to the articular surfaces in the knee joint, especially the thigh-bone condyles and the back of the kneecap. Sometimes there is simply softening of the articular cartilage; sometimes pieces of articular cartilage break away from the underlying bone. There may be quite big fragments floating around the knee joint cavity. The condition is called osteochondritis dissecans.

The damage shows up on X-rays. It can occur as the result of bad knocks to the knee which cause minor fractures in the affected bone surface. There may be other problems in the knee, such as kneecap pain syndrome or Osgood-Schlatter's condition.

Osteochondritis dissecans can be present in the knee without causing any symptoms, but it can cause mild swelling, aching and a curious clicking feeling on certain movements. If it is causing problems, surgery may be needed to remove any larger floating bone fragments, or possibly to re-attach them to the underlying bone. If the patient is in a lot of pain, the knee may be immobilized in a plaster cast for four to eight weeks. In most cases, the problem settles simply with remedial exercises and rest from pain-causing activities.

Soft-tissue injuries

7

CARTILAGE INJURIES

A tear of the knee's soft cartilage (meniscus) is usually a traumatic injury which can happen if the knee is bent and twisted awkwardly, or forced backwards or sideways when the joint is straight. Most often the tear happens because one (or sometimes both) of the cartilages is trapped in the wrong position between the shin-bone and the thigh-bone. The cartilage can split across its width in a transverse tear, or down its length in a longitudinal tear. The tear can be partial or total. Other types of damage can happen to the cartilage, including the formation of cysts on the cartilage due to trauma or friction.

One or both cartilages can be injured separately, together, or in conjunction with other tissues in the knee, such as the cruciate ligaments, medial or lateral ligaments, articular cartilage surfaces or joint capsule. The degree of damage depends on the severity and direction of the traumatic force applied to the knee. As the medial cartilage is attached

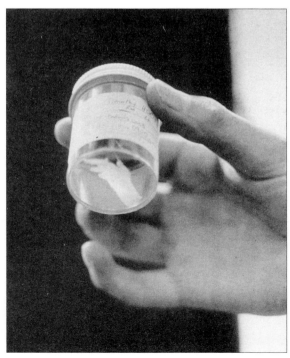

A torn cartilage removed

to the medial ligament, injuring both together is relatively common.

Hereditary factors can make cartilage injury more likely. Some children are born with so-called discoid cartilages, which are rounder and more solid than normal. Because the central edges are thickened, they can more easily be damaged by pressure from the bone ends forming the knee, especially in active children.

If the knee and its cartilages are healthy and stable, it takes quite a degree of force to cause a cartilage tear. However, if this is not the case, the cartilages can be torn much more easily, sometimes without any obvious traumatic accident. Cartilage injuries are more likely to happen if there have been previous injuries to the knee or its muscles without a return to full strength, stability and mobility. If a minor cartilage tear goes undetected, it can lead to a more disabling tear later. If one knee has been injured previously and the other overloaded as a result, the cartilages on the previously sound knee can suffer.

The cartilages can also suffer from attritional damage through overuse pressures. With age, they can become fragile and worn through repetitive pressures caused by activities like long-distance running. The full-squat movement under maximum load, as in heavy weightlifting and powerlifting, can over time be too much for the cartilages to withstand. Obesity can cause overload on the cartilages when the obese person stands for long periods or walks any distance. Any movement limitation in the knee which prevents it from bending or straightening fully can mean that the central parts of the cartilages are subjected to excessive repetitive loading during walking or running.

Who gets cartilage injuries?

Cartilage tears can happen to anyone at any age. The injury is very common among soccer, rugby and American football players. It can happen during a blocked tackle or a twisting movement when the boot studs have got stuck in the ground. Forcing the knee into an exaggerated position of full bending and twisting can split a cartilage. This can happen to breast-stroke swimmers who apply too much pressure when they do the 'frog-sitting' stretch in which they kneel down and sit back on their haunches with their feet alongside their hips. Cossack dancing or doing the Limbo, Twist or Charleston can cause cartilage tears. People who crouch or kneel and then get up awkwardly, as can happen when gardening, carpet-laying or simply picking something up from the floor, can trap and tear a cartilage, especially if their leg muscles are weak. Compressive movements after the knees have been held still can lead to cartilage tear, as when a bus driver jumps down from the cab on to straight legs after sitting with the knees bent for a long period.

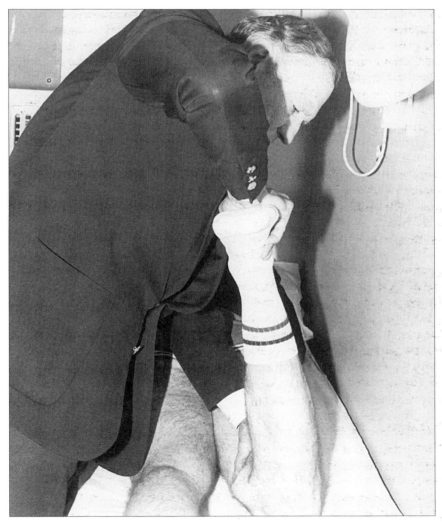

The Apley 'grind' test for cartilage tear

How cartilage injuries are diagnosed

The main indicators suggesting cartilage injury are the history of how the problem started, the type of pain and the functional deficits which interfere with the patient's normal activities. There are many external tests in which the knee is manipulated with the aim of identifying cartilage damage. These tests are usually named after their originators, such as Apley's, Bragard's, Helfet's, McMurray's, Merke's, O'Donoghue's, Payr's and Steinmann's. They are not foolproof. While a positive test can confirm cartilage damage, negative findings do not necessarily prove the opposite, so the patient is usually sent for investigations such as an MRI scan. If cartilage damage seems extremely likely, arthroscopy may be performed with the dual purpose of confirming the injury and operating on the damage.

How cartilage injuries are treated

If the injured semilunar cartilage is not hindering the knee or causing any obvious problems, the knee can be rehabilitated conservatively. Provided you reach full recovery with no functional deficits or muscle imbalance, and can bend and straighten the knee fully, you can safely return to sports. However, if at any stage the torn part of the semilunar cartilage is catching and blocking the knee's normal movements, it is unlikely that the situation can improve without surgery. Every time that the knee catches painfully or locks, damage is probably occurring on the articular cartilage of the joint, which can lead to long-term problems of wear-and-tear degeneration (osteoarthritis).

Attitudes to surgery for the semilunar cartilages have changed considerably because of improvements in diagnostic and surgical techniques. When surgery had to involve opening the knee through a scar, many surgeons preferred to wait and see whether the problem would settle, rather than subjecting the knee to further trauma, whereas others still considered it better to operate sooner rather than later. Now that arthroscopy has made cartilage operations relatively safe and non-invasive using micro-surgery, it is almost certainly better for the troublesome cartilage to be operated on as quickly as possible. The surgeon may repair the torn cartilage by stitching it together, cut out a cyst or torn part in a partial meniscectomy, or remove the damaged cartilage completely (total meniscectomy), according to the extent and nature of the injury.

How long does it take to recover from cartilage injuries?

Without surgery, recovery from minor injuries involving the semilunar cartilages can take between about four and twelve weeks of rehabilitation. After arthroscopic surgery, recovery is apparently quick, and it may be tempting to try to return to active sports after two to three weeks, especially for the serious or professional sports player. However, this causes a grave risk of longer-term damage in the joint, whether the patient is a child or an adult. Sports activities may become increasingly limited over time by after-effects such as weakness and giving way as the joint surfaces degenerate progressively.

It is extremely important for the patient to make a full recovery from the injury and the surgery before returning to physically stressful activities. The knee needs to recover its full co-ordination mechanisms and proprioception in order to function properly and to prevent re-injury or secondary injury. For the child and adult patient alike, I allow about six weeks of progressive rehabilitation post-operatively, to make sure that the knee has recovered fully before allowing a return to sports involving running, jumping, twisting and turning, kicking or contact.

The long-term results following open surgery for cartilage injuries were generally poor, with many patients suffering arthritic changes in the operated joint years later. Arthroscopic surgery should show much better results in the future, but this may well depend on the quality of the rehabilitation after-care.

CRUCIATE LIGAMENT TEARS

A severe wrench to the knee can strain or tear one or both of the cruciate ligaments in the centre of the joint, with or without causing damage to other structures such as the semilunar cartilages. The anterior cruciate ligament is injured more frequently than the posterior cruciate. In very rare cases, both cruciate ligaments are injured together. Either can be torn or strained when the knee is forcibly twisted or hyperextended, especially with the foot fixed on the ground. The posterior cruciate ligament is very likely to be injured if the thigh-bone glides forwards forcibly over the shin-bone with the knee bent and the foot on the ground.

Cruciate ligament injuries are a special risk in skiing and in contact sports like rugby, soccer, American football and hockey. They can also happen without contact in sports like tennis and netball, when the injury may be attritional and perhaps caused by inappropriate shoes which grip too hard or slip on the hard court surfaces. Non-sporting accidents, such as a bad fall or a car or motorcycle accident, can also cause cruciate ligament injuries. In pre-teenagers, injury to the anterior cruciate ligament often causes an avulsion fracture of its attachment to the shin-bone, and is very often accompanied by injury to the medial ligament. In youngsters, posterior cruciate ligament tears are very rare, but when they do happen they usually involve an avulsion fracture from the attachment on the thigh-bone. In teenagers, the cruciate ligaments may be more vulnerable to tears during the growth spurts, especially if the teenager is very tall and slim, with relatively weak musculature supporting the elongated bones.

At the moment of injury there may be severe pain, or surprisingly little. There may be a 'popping' or snapping sound, and a sensation of a tear

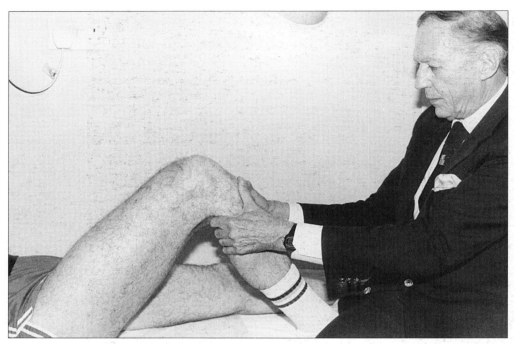

The anterior drawer test for anterior cruciate insufficiency

deep inside the knee, but it is not always obvious. Sometimes the victim feels well enough to carry on skiing, running or playing, but the knee quickly feels unstable and painful. It usually swells up immediately, although the amount of swelling may be slight. Later on, laxity due to cruciate damage can make the knee feel vulnerable in certain situations, especially when turning slightly sideways over the injured leg while standing up.

How cruciate ligament injuries are diagnosed

The history of how the injury happened, the pattern of pain and the feeling of instability are pointers indicating cruciate ligament damage. External manipulative tests include the pivot shift, anterior drawer, Lachman's anterior drawer, Noyes's flexion-rotation drawer, Slocum's, MacIntosh's, Losee's, posterior drawer, posterior tibial sag, posterolateral drawer, and reverse pivot shift. These tests reveal the degree of instability in the various directions of the knee's movements, and they may then be confirmed with investigations such as an MRI scan.

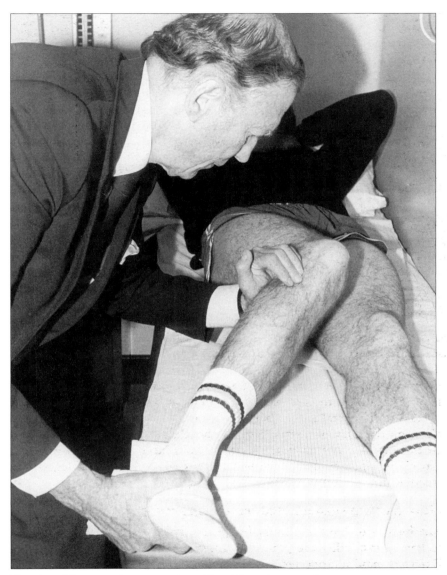

The pivot shift test to show antero-lateral instability

How cruciate ligament injuries are treated

Diagnosis of the cruciate tear or strain may not be immediate, if the injury does not appear to be major. Sometimes damage to other tissues may mask the cruciate injury, or make it seem a lesser priority even if it is recognized. Treatment for the injured cruciate ligament depends largely on the surgeon. There may be an immediate decision to operate to repair or reconstruct the ligament if it is badly torn and the surgeon feels surgery will be successful. If there is multiple damage inside the knee, perhaps to a cartilage as well as a cruciate ligament, the surgeon may opt to deal with the cartilage and leave the cruciate ligament to be treated conservatively. Conservative treatment may be the option chosen if the ligament is stretched or only partly torn, or if the patient is not particularly active in

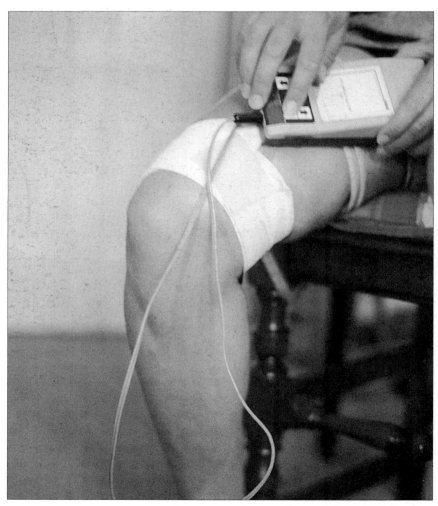

Self-help electrical muscle stimulation for the hamstrings, especially biceps femoris, may be part of conservative or post-operative rehabilitation following cruciate ligament injury

sports. Conservative treatment involves strengthening the knee's controlling muscles and working at co-ordination exercises, especially involving the hamstring muscles. It takes time for the programme to have its effect, so the patient has to commit at least six months to the remedial exercise regime.

In some cases the knee seems to recover well following the injury, except that it occasionally feels unstable, as if it is about to give way. This happens in very specific situations, for instance when the patient is

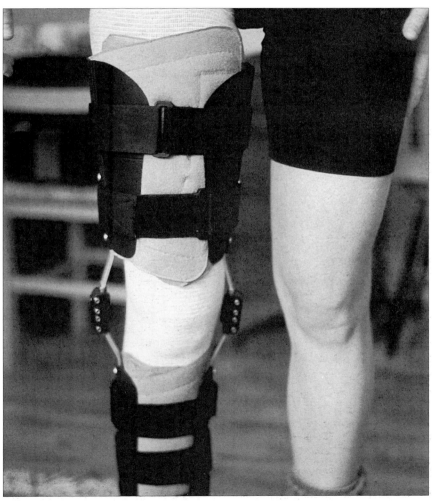

A brace to protect the knee after cruciate ligament repair surgery

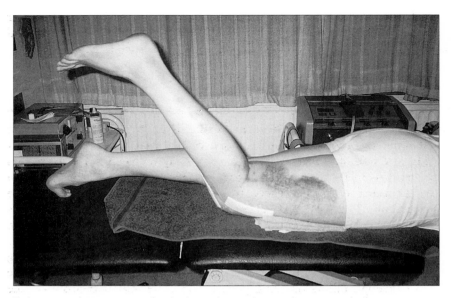

Early stage active movement for the hamstrings against gravity, one week after surgery to repair a torn anterior cruciate ligament. The thigh is supported for comfort, and no part of the movement is forced through pain

standing up and turns slightly to one side. In this case, the patient should be referred back to the surgeon, or sent for a second opinion, as surgery may be the best option for correcting this.

Surgery for cruciate ligament damage is complex, and many different techniques are used, according to the nature of the injury and the surgeon's preference and level of expertise. If the ligament has torn away (avulsed) its bony attachment, it may be re-attached with a screw. If the ligament itself is broken it may be stitched back together, or reinforced with tissue taken from another structure like the patellar tendon. Various materials have been used to create artificial replacements for the cruciate ligaments. In some operations, which are probably used less often now than previously, the damaged ligament is not touched, but the joint mechanics are stabilized through tightening up other structures, for instance at the outer side of the knee in the case of damage to the anterior cruciate.

Following surgery, the patient may be kept in bed for a period, or may be allowed up using crutches, with the operated leg protected in a plaster cast or, more usually nowadays, in a wadded bandage. Remedial exercises are started straight away and functional activities are gradually increased. Full recovery takes up to a year or more, and the remedial exercises have to be maintained throughout the recovery period and preferably long afterwards. Even after full recovery, the patient may use a specially fitted knee brace for extra protection in high-risk sports such as skiing.

MEDIAL LIGAMENT INJURIES

The medial collateral ligament on the inner side of the knee can be injured traumatically by a sudden violent force which opens up that side of the joint. The ligament may be totally or partly torn, sometimes together with the medial semilunar cartilage which is attached to it. In children and young teenagers, the medial ligament is less likely to be injured in this kind of accident than the shin-bone where it is attached, as this is a vulnerable growth area. However, very young children have been known to tear the medial ligament.

Traumatic medial ligament injuries can happen when someone is doing the sideways splits and overbalances or is pushed, or from twisting the knee through falling or being pushed while the foot is blocked on the ground and the rest of the body is turning outwards. Medial ligament injuries can happen easily in any contact sport such as soccer, American football, rugby, tae kwon do or judo.

Overuse strains of the medial ligament can happen if the knee is repetitively bent and twisted awkwardly. This can be an effect of intensive breast-stroke swimming, so it is often called 'breast-stroker's knee'. It can also happen because of poor technique in karate kicking movements, or overdoing the stepping and twisting movements in an aerobic step class.

When the medial ligament is completely torn there is usually severe pain over the inner side of the knee, and the joint feels unstable, as though it 'comes apart'. Stress X-rays may be taken in which pressure is put against that side of the knee (technically valgus stress) in order to show the gap in the joint. Stress X-rays are especially likely to be taken in the case of a child, as any fractures in the growth areas of the bones will show up. The orthopaedic surgeon may decide to operate to mend the ligament, or the leg may be protected in a plaster cast for several weeks. If there is a bone fracture, it may be necessary to stabilize it through operation.

Whatever the treatment, during the active recovery phase the ligament is likely to be painful on straightening and bending the knee. It can be treated with ice, massage, and perhaps electrotherapy techniques, of which I normally choose diadynamic currents. I sometimes use ultrasound for pain relief on adult patients, but never on children. Soft-tissue manipulations may help to restore full movement in the knee. It is vital to

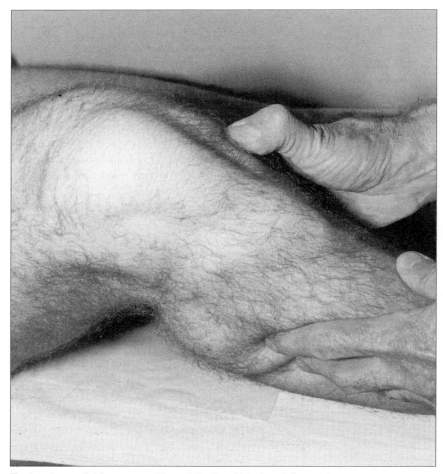

Testing the medial ligament and inner joint line (right knee) for tenderness

regain good balance between the vastus medialis obliquus, adductor muscles and hamstrings as well as full co-ordination in all the knee movements. Sometimes the full squat movement is recovered slowly, but in a few cases squatting can be painless from an early stage of recovery.

Full recovery from a severe medial ligament injury usually takes at least three months. A more minor strain can take as long, although it may recover within four to six weeks. If bone fractures are also involved, the recovery phase may be much more protracted.

PES ANSERINUS STRAIN

The pes anserinus, the group of tendons which attaches to the top of the inner side of the shin-bone, can be strained in association with any injury which stresses the inner side of the knee. Strain can also be caused by poor posture, especially sitting with the knee slightly twisted for long periods. The injury causes an irritating point of pain just below the knee, especially on movements which involve a very slight twist. The pain can become very severe at times, although this tends not to last. In walking, the pain may be felt most acutely when the foot is off the ground as the leg comes forward. The pain can inhibit normal knee movement, weakening vastus medialis obliquus function.

Treatment for pes anserinus strain usually consists of ice applications to the tender area, perhaps gentle massage, and particular attention to exercises which stabilize the knee in the straight position. If knee-straightening movements hurt, ice is used to reduce the pain while the exercises are done.

LATERAL LIGAMENT INJURIES

The lateral ligament is rarely injured on its own. Strains over the outer side of the knee usually cause injury to the arcuate ligament and popliteus tendon as well as the lateral ligament. In severe injuries there may be bony avulsion fractures. Sometimes the outer semilunar cartilage is involved.

The typical cause of injury to the structures on the outer side of the knee is a strain which opens up that side, as in a sideways fall while skiing, or a football tackle against the outer side of the foot or leg. The pain is localized to that side of the knee. There is restriction of movement and there may be swelling. Any movement which presses the knee outwards is painful, especially if the patient bends the knee and twists the hip outwards, as in sitting cross-legged on the floor.

Surgery may be needed for the more severe type of injury, especially if the semilunar cartilage is damaged. More often injuries to the outer side of the knee can be treated successfully with bandaging, taping or a cast to protect the joint from painful movements, and by progressive remedial exercises.

ILIOTIBIAL TRACT INJURIES

The iliotibial tract (band) on the outer side of the thigh can be injured traumatically if the knee is forcibly wrenched sideways. This can happen in a bad fall on to the outer side of the body, or in a tackle which forces the foot inwards. The injury may tear the band itself, or pull away the iliotibial tract's bony attachment points at the top of the shin-bone or the fibula. In a severe injury, other structures may be injured as well, especially the lateral ligament of the knee, and sometimes one of the semilunar cartilages or cruciate ligaments.

Treatment depends on the severity of the injury. The orthopaedic surgeon has to decide on the priorities if there is major disruption inside the knee. If the iliotibial tract alone is injured, it is usually treated by protection in a cast or knee brace until the pain has subsided, followed by a course of remedial exercises to restore stability and functional movement.

Iliotibial tract friction syndrome is an overuse injury associated with running, cycling, cross-country skiing and walking. It causes a very specific pain pattern. The pain is felt just above the outer side of the knee, and comes on after a certain amount of the activity, for instance after about a mile of running. At first it may wear off if the activity is continued, but if the problem develops, the pain becomes too severe to continue, although it usually stops quickly after the end of the activity and does not interfere with other types of sport or everyday activities.

The pain pattern is usually caused by irritation or inflammation in the iliotibial tract itself or the bursa which lies under the tract. This can come on as the result of altered mechanics affecting the outer side of the knee, perhaps through running on camber, or using shoes or boots which tip the feet too far outwards into supination and inversion. Over-pronation at the foot coupled with a slight inwards twist of the shin-bone during walking and running can also cause irritation. Hip problems can affect the knee mechanics of runners, cyclists and cross-country skiers.

There may be a swollen 'lump' at the painful point, which can feel extremely tender when it is pressed while the knee is bent to an angle of about 30 degrees. The iliotibial tract is usually tight. The flexibility of the outer thigh can be tested with Ober's test: the patient lies on the unaffected side with the leg bent; the practitioner holds the injured leg with the knee bent to a right angle and gently lowers it to see how far down behind the other leg it reaches.

Once the problem has been diagnosed, it is usually treated conservatively. Besides using electrical muscle stimulation for vastus medialis obliquus (see p.147), I treat the problem with ice, massage and diadynamic currents for the tender area, with the knee supported in a slightly bent position. If the hip is involved in the problem, I treat it with manual mobilizing techniques. Apart from the basic remedial knee exercises, the patient has to do stretching exercises for the outer thigh. Shoes are corrected or replaced, if necessary. If poor foot mechanics are implicated, the patient may be referred to a podiatrist for custom-made insoles (orthotics).

When the problem is slight, recovery can be very quick, needing only a few days, but if it is more severe it can last several weeks. During the recovery period the patient has to avoid pain-causing activities, but is usually able to do at least some running, cycling, cross-country skiing or walking, especially if the mechanics can be altered, for instance by using different shoes, correcting the pattern of movement from the hip, or running sideways and backwards at intervals.

If the problem does not improve with conservative treatment, the doctor may inject the painful spot, or, as a last resort, the orthopaedic surgeon may operate to clear out the inflamed area. Afterwards, the patient follows a rehabilitation programme and then gradually returns to normal sports activities.

BURSITIS

Like the bursa under the iliotibial tract, the other bursae around the knee can become inflamed, swollen and painful. This is usually the result of injury or an inflammatory condition. Direct trauma such as a blow on to the bursa can cause an immediate swelling which is usually contained and egg-shaped. If the bursa splits, the excess fluid spreads into the surrounding tissues and can cause bruising over a much wider area. Bursitis can also arise through friction, especially if the knee is not operating mechanically as smoothly as it should, perhaps as the result of some previous injury or through faulty foot mechanics. Repetitive activities like long-distance running or constant pressure through crouching or kneeling for long periods can cause irritation and inflammation in the soft tissues.

When inflammation happens in the prepatellar bursa under the skin over the front of the kneecap, it is called 'housemaid's knee'. A similar swollen lump at the back of the knee is a Baker's cyst, which can be formed from one of the bursae, or sometimes the gastrocnemius bursa under the inner head of the muscle joins up with the popliteus bursa and the knee joint capsule to form a very prominent swelling. Localized inflammation is also relatively common in the pes anserinus bursa

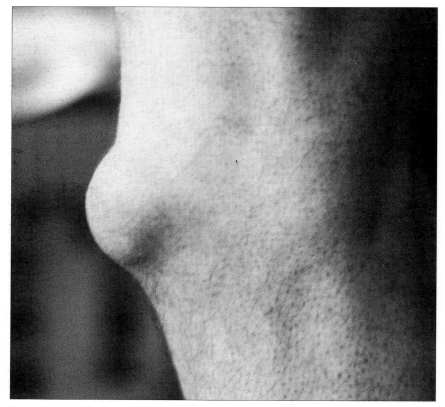

Prepatellar bursitis ('housemaid's knee')

between the tendons and the medial ligament, the suprapatellar bursa under the quadriceps tendon just above the kneecap, and the bursa under the semimembranosus tendon at the inner side of the back of the knee.

A swollen or inflamed bursa can be painless or it can cause localized symptoms, often feeling sore and hot. Sometimes it mimics the symptoms of other knee problems. Most often, bursitis interferes with the knee's full movement. If it is painful there is usually muscle inhibition and weakness.

Treatment for any bursitis depends on the cause of the problem and the extent to which it is interfering with the knee's normal function. In extreme cases, the excess fluid may be drained out of the bursa, or the bursa itself may be removed surgically, but it is quite common for the problem to recur after these procedures. In most cases, for post-operative or conservative treatment, the patient is referred for physiotherapy. Ice, massage and possibly electrotherapy may be used to help reduce the localized swelling. The priority is to restore full movement and stability in

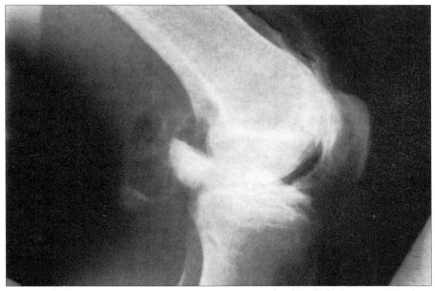

Baker's cyst behind the knee (left side of picture) shown up on an arthrogram

the knee. Self-help measures include ice applications, perhaps arnica compresses, and daily remedial exercises. Any painful or irritating repetitive activities should be avoided. It may help to wear protective knee pads if the painful area tends to get knocked.

INFRAPATELLAR FAT PAD INJURY

The infrapatellar fat pad, which lies between the patellar tendon and the synovial membrane of the knee, is a very common site of pain through direct trauma, such as a blow or a fall on the front of the knee. This type of injury is common in roller-blading and skateboarding, especially if protective knee pads are not used. It can happen in sports like American football, if the knee pads are poorly fitted. Before seat belts were widely used in cars, injury to the fat pads in car accidents, known as 'dashboard knee', was commonplace. The fat pads are more easily injured in hyperextending knees, because the bones of the knee tend to impinge on them. In females, fluid retention due to hormonal activity or changes, such as premenstrually, can make the infrapatellar fat pads in both knees swell so that they become painful through compression.

Sometimes, pain from infrapatellar fat pad problems seems very similar to that of kneecap pain syndrome, so the diagnosis has to be made with care. The fat pad may also be enlarged as the result of a semilunar cartilage tear, in which case surgical treatment of the cartilage usually leads to relief of the pain and swelling in the fat pad. It is quite common for the infrapatellar fat pad to become swollen and slightly sore following any surgical procedures for the knee, but this usually settles quickly in the course of rehabilitation treatment. Pain from the inflamed infrapatellar fat pad is usually at its worst when the knee is straightened fully. The fat pad looks swollen on one or both sides of the patellar tendon, and feels tender to touch and sometimes warm.

In chronic or severe cases, surgery may be needed to remove damaged tissue from the fat pad. Post-operatively or conservatively, the fat pad can be treated with ice applications and gentle massage. Particular attention has to be paid to restoring vastus medialis obliquus function with remedial exercises, usually in conjunction with electrical muscle stimulation.

SYNOVIAL PLICA SYNDROME

The synovial lining of the knee may have folds, called plicae, in it due to incomplete development. These are attached around the knee above and to the outer side of the kneecap and along the inner (medial) side of the thigh-bone knuckle to the inner part of the infrapatellar fat pad. The folds can become inflamed and thickened through faulty mechanics or trauma around the knee, causing impingement and pain in the knee. This problem is usually called the plica syndrome.

Once a plica has been diagnosed, it may be removed surgically if it fails to respond to conservative treatment. Following surgery, there is always very marked inhibition of the vastus medialis obliquus muscle, so this is the priority for rehabilitation. Recovery of the VMO can take weeks or even months, and has to be completed before the knee can be stressed in normal or sporting weightbearing activities.

MUSCLE AND TENDON INJURIES AROUND THE KNEE

Injury to any of the muscles and tendons around the knee has an effect on knee function. The movements of the knee are inevitably impaired, muscle imbalance is created around the knee, and there is also imbalance between the injured leg and the other. If these functional deficits are not corrected, they can cause problems in the longer term.

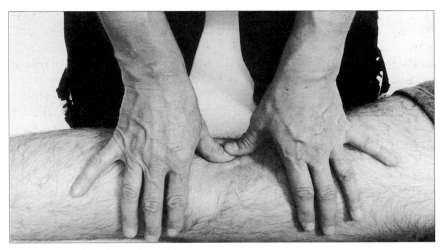

Palpating one of the hamstring tendons

The muscles and tendons can be torn or strained traumatically through a sudden direct blow or fall, as can happen in any contact sport, or by a fall from a ladder. They can also fail dramatically for little or no apparent reason, as in the sprinter's sudden hamstring tear. Overuse injuries to the muscles or tendons can arise from factors like fatigue, unbalanced training schedules, ill-prepared sports activities and poor postural habits.

If one or more of the quadriceps muscles are injured, the knee cannot bend fully, and the controlling mechanism to straighten it is weakened. This is especially inhibiting if the vastus medialis muscle is involved in the injury, causing loss of control of the kneecap from the inner side and failure of the knee's locking-out mechanism when it is fully straightened. When rectus femoris, the longest of the quadriceps muscles, is injured, the hip is affected as well as the knee, so both joints may become fixed in the flexed position. Injury to the adductor muscles on the inner side of the thigh usually has an effect on the vastus medialis, even if the latter is not directly involved in the injury. When the adductors are tightened and weakened through injury, they draw the hip inwards and tend to pull the knee into a slightly bent and twisted position.

Hamstring injuries create shortening on the back of the thigh and knee, drawing the knee into the bent position, and pulling the pelvis into a backward tilt. Inefficiency in the hamstrings is a particular handicap for sprinting and jumping, and can lead to longer-term problems in the knee, hip or lower back. Being two-joint muscles, the hamstrings are especially vulnerable to injury. If the person's water intake is inadequate they tend to cramp very easily when they are contracted, especially when the knee is

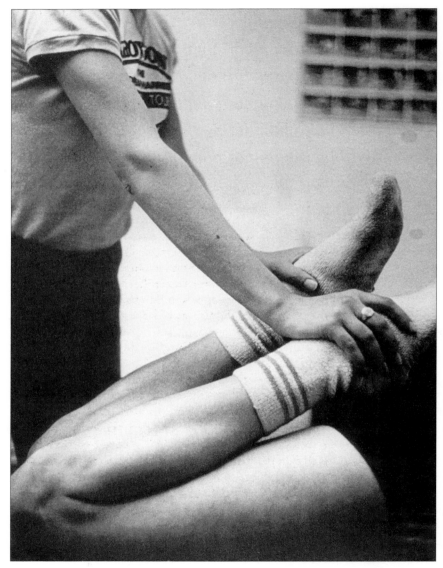

Limited flexibility in the left thigh following a quadriceps muscle tear must be corrected to prevent secondary knee problems

bent in the stomach-lying position, and this can be a factor in overuse strains.

Because of the attachment of the gastrocnemius tendons behind the knee, calf muscle injuries can also cause tightness at the back of the knee, especially if the tendons themselves are strained or torn.

There are many different ways of treating muscle and tendon injuries, including anti-inflammatory drugs, and various forms of electrotherapy. In the early stages of a traumatic tear, treatment has to be carefully limited, usually to ice or hot-and-cold applications, very gentle movements and stretching exercises within pain limits, and possibly light massage around the area. Any more invasive treatments to the torn area are likely to increase internal bleeding and swelling. In the case of the quadriceps muscles in particular, this creates a risk of bone formation within the muscle, which is called myositis ossificans.

For all muscle or tendon injuries I use manual therapy, progressive exercises and, as soon as possible, electrical muscle stimulation to regain efficient muscle activity. Full sporting activities should not be allowed until the injured area has regained its flexibility, strength and co-ordination. Controlled stretching exercises should remain a daily routine, and should be repeated before and after any other type of exercise or sport.

PATELLAR TENDON INJURIES

The patellar tendon can be torn if the quadriceps muscles exert excessive force on the tendon by contracting especially hard to straighten the knee from the bent position. This can happen when an opponent blocks a kick in soccer, American football or rugby, or through squatting with too heavy a load in weightlifting or powerlifting. A complete tear may happen more easily if the patellar tendon has been treated for previous strains with injections into the central part of the tendon. Taking anabolic steroid drugs to increase muscle strength and enhance performance can also weaken the substance of the tendon and make it more fragile.

How patellar tendon injuries happen

The traumatic patellar tendon tear can happen in children, although up to the mid-teens they are more likely to suffer an avulsion fracture of the tibial tubercle. The injury is more common in adults and older people. As it is very disabling, it usually needs immediate surgical repair, followed by a period of protection in a plaster cast. After removal of the plaster, treatment is needed to help restore mobility in the knee and stability to the muscles. Full recovery can take several months.

Overuse strains to the patellar tendon can result from repeated movements which stress the tendon and its attachment points on the tibial tubercle and the lower pole of the kneecap. Patellar tendinitis, which is often called 'jumper's knee', usually arises from intensive practice of activities like high jumping, volleyball, basketball, soccer, hopping and bounding training and hill running. It can happen at any age, although in young teenagers there is more likely to be damage to the tibial tubercle or the lower pole of the kneecap than to the tendon. Previous Osgood-Schlatter's condition, inflexibility in the quadriceps mechanism following previous injury to the muscles or the knee, malalignment of the kneecap or excessive pronation at the foot can all contribute to patellar tendon overuse injury.

The pain pattern in patellar tendon injuries

The typical features are tenderness over the patellar tendon, localized pain on squatting, running, jumping, kneeling and walking up and down stairs, and sometimes swelling over the front of the knee. There may also be pain when the knee is straightened out fully. If the tendon is strained where it is attached to the lower pole of the kneecap, there may be a spot over the bone which is excruciatingly tender on direct pressure, indicating damage to the bone itself or sometimes the formation of tiny cysts. This is called Sinding-Larsen-Johansson's 'disease' or condition, and it is especially common among teenagers, although it can happen at any age.

In mild cases, the pain may be felt only after activity. Later on, the pain can come on at the start of the causative sport or activity, easing as the patient warms up, only to recur towards the end, getting progressively more noticeable each time the painful movements are repeated. Eventually, the pain becomes too severe to permit movements which stress the patellar tendon.

Treatment for patellar tendon injuries

Treatment depends on the severity of the condition. Rest from painful activities is a must. Ice, anti-inflammatory drugs, supportive braces and various forms of electrotherapy have all been used with good effect to reduce the discomfort. I usually treat the tendon with soft-tissue manipulation, and ask the patient to use ice and perhaps gentle self-massage for the tendon on a daily basis. I use electrical muscle stimulation for vastus medialis obliquus, especially if there is pain on full knee extension, as it is vital to prevent the loss of the extension mechanism. If the tendon is not too tender, especially in the later stages of recovery, I

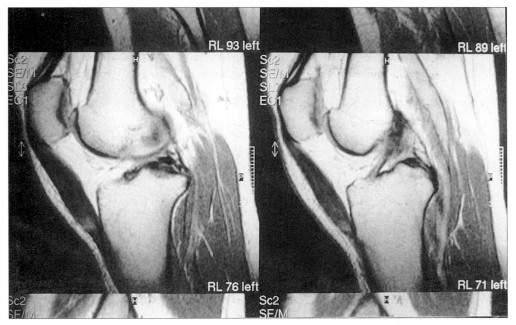

Sections of the patellar tendon and knee bones shown on an MRI scan of a patient with chronic patellar tendon injury

may also use electrical stimulation directly over it, with the knee supported slightly bent, to promote efficient extension movement using the tendon's activity. The patient has to do very gentle quadriceps stretching exercises regularly, and progressive strengthening work.

If the pain in the tendon is severe and investigations show bone damage or cyst formation, surgery may be needed to clear the debris: technically this is called debridement. It may also be necessary to reinforce the tendon, which may be done by simply putting a stitch into it. Sometimes, the surgery is done under local anaesthetic. Following surgery, the knee is protected for a few days, but weightbearing and gentle exercises are started immediately, and progressed according to the patient's pain levels.

Recovery from patellar tendon injuries of all kinds is complete when the patient can do all normal activities and squat fully and symmetrically. Kneeling is likely to remain painful for a long time, sometimes indefinitely after good functional recovery has been achieved. A minor patellar tendon injury can recover quickly, but more often the problem takes anything from three to twelve months.

Practitioners, diagnosis and assessment

8

WHICH PRACTITIONER?

Most knee problems do not just go away of their own accord. They need treatment. Even in the case of young children's injuries and pains, which may seem to heal readily in the pre-teen years, it is always wiser to have the problem assessed by a specialist, to avoid later consequences arising out of a residual weakness.

The role of the practitioner is to analyse the problem, identify its cause,

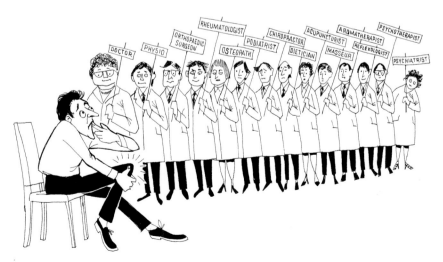

Choosing the right practitioner can seem difficult

establish the diagnosis with as much certainty as possible, and institute a treatment and rehabilitation strategy. The practitioner may need to refer some patients to a specialist. Teamwork and good co-operation between practitioners are essential for the comprehensive care of knee problems.

Various practitioners may be involved in the diagnosis, assessment and treatment, according to the cause and nature of the knee problem. Any serious injury is likely to be treated by an orthopaedic surgeon. An injury which does not need surgery may be referred to an orthopaedic doctor. A rheumatologist may be consulted if a knee problem is likely to be related to an inflammatory condition or disease, or an infection. If the nerve systems in the leg seem to have been disrupted, a neurologist may be involved. In situations where the patient needs drug therapy but prefers not to use pharmaceutical products, the family doctor may refer the patient to a homoeopathic doctor, who uses naturally occurring substances to stimulate the body's healing systems. Most of the 'hands-on' treatment of knee injuries is done by paramedical practitioners such as physiotherapists.

Every practitioner has a fairly well-defined area of practice and expertise, although there are areas of overlap between some professions. You need to be aware of what different practitioners are qualified to do, and what their limitations are in order to understand why you are being referred to a particular practitioner or whether a practitioner you have chosen is appropriate.

FINDING THE RIGHT PROFESSIONAL

You risk being seriously confused, and probably misled, if you go about finding a practitioner to treat your problem in the wrong way. If you take advice from friends or acquaintances who have seemingly had the same problem, you may end up consulting the wrong kind of specialist for your problem. If you consult several different practitioners without reference to each other you are likely to receive conflicting opinions and advice. If you try to interpret, alter or add to any professional advice you have received, or, worse still, mix different types of treatment on your own initiative, you will probably just make your problem worse. Although you need to be informed about what might be wrong with your knee and the possible ways of dealing with it, it is a mistake to try to read technical articles if you do not fully understand them. The Internet has made a lot of very specialized technical information widely available, so it can be tempting to seek answers to problems by 'surfing' through apparently relevant subject matter. This can be a recipe for confusion or depression.

If you need advice on any aspect of your knee problem, you should ask a professionally qualified person. The best starting point is the general practitioner (GP or family doctor), who has an overall view of your medical history and past injuries. The GP is well placed to decide whether the problem should be assessed by an orthopaedic surgeon, rheumatologist, or another type of specialist, or whether it can be treated conservatively in the first instance by a medical or paramedical practitioner. Investigations such as X-rays, scans or blood tests may be organized by the family doctor immediately or at a later stage, or they may be left to the discretion of the specialist.

PARAMEDICAL PRACTITIONERS

Various paramedical practitioners may be involved in the conservative treatment of knee problems, depending on the situation.

In the majority of cases, knee problems need rehabilitation treatment, which should be under the guidance of a qualified practitioner such as a physiotherapist (physical therapist) or athletic trainer. The qualified physiotherapist is trained to apply a variety of physical treatments for different kinds of patients, including manual therapy, electrotherapy, hydrotherapy and, most importantly, exercise therapy. Athletic training, which is an American professional qualification, covers a similar range of treatment modalities, as applied to sports players.

Osteopaths or chiropractors, who are specialized in manipulative techniques, may treat knee problems, especially if the patient also has symptoms stemming from a back problem. An acupuncturist can help to relieve pain and to improve some types of defects affecting the circulatory system. Reflexologists, who apply energy through the healing meridians of the foot, can also help with pain relief and circulatory improvement. If custom-made knee supports are needed, an orthotist or occupational therapist may supply and fit them. If foot problems are a significant part of a knee problem, a podiatrist or chiropodist may fit customized foot supports, which are called orthotics, although the term also applies to supportive appliances for other parts of the body. The patient with weight problems or food intolerance reactions may need help from a dietician or nutritionist.

In Britain and many other countries you can consult paramedical practitioners such as chartered physiotherapists and osteopaths without reference to your general practitioner. It is always important to know that the practitioner you choose is properly qualified, and preferably covered by professional indemnity insurance. This is necessary if you go for private treatment and wish to recover the fees under a medical insurance scheme. It is also advisable as a safety measure, to ensure that you receive appropriate treatment from a practitioner who is ethically recognized. If in doubt, do not just accept an impressive-looking row of letters after the name as proof: ask the practitioner what his or her qualifications are, and if there is still doubt, check his or her registration with the appropriate professional body.

DIAGNOSIS OF KNEE PROBLEMS

The diagnosis is the definition of exactly what is wrong with your knee. As the first steps towards establishing the diagnosis the practitioner listens to and analyses your description of the problem, and then examines you physically. These two elements are called the assessment, and they may be sufficient to establish a working diagnosis on the basis of which a suitable treatment strategy can be set up. There are many manual tests which may show whether there is instability or an internal derangement like a torn cartilage or ruptured cruciate ligament. Done skilfully, they can be useful guides, but these external tests are still notoriously imprecise when compared to the various scanning techniques and arthroscopy, so they can be misleading to both patient and practitioner. For more conclusive evidence, specialist investigations such as blood tests, X-rays and scans are needed.

Depending on the type of problem, a completely accurate diagnosis can only be established by the doctor or surgeon. If the physiotherapist or another paramedical practitioner is the first contact, the aim of the assessment is simply to establish which type of treatment might be appropriate for reducing the symptoms, and whether any of the basic remedial exercises can be done safely without causing pain.

The precise diagnosis of any condition or internal damage is not necessarily essential to the process of functional correction. However, when assessing a problem knee, the physiotherapist or other paramedical practitioner needs to be able to recognize whether there is a likelihood of internal damage. After a known injury, swelling in the knee, certain patterns of pain, movement inhibition and other symptoms such as locking indicate the likelihood of internal damage. If these symptoms persist without diminishing during a conservative rehabilitation treatment programme, the physiotherapist may recommend that you see your general practitioner and discuss the possibility of being referred to an orthopaedic consultant. If there is no history of injury, food intolerance (see p.46) is usually taken into account. If the source of the symptoms is unclear, you may be referred back to your general practitioner in case there is an infection or inflammatory disease that should be investigated.

WHAT YOU NEED TO TELL THE PRACTITIONER

It is the patient's duty to help the practitioner understand the problem, and it is the practitioner's duty to encourage and help the patient to tell the story of the problem as fully as possible and to take note of all the relevant facts. The process may seem laborious, but time spent taking an accurate history is time well spent, and can save patient and practitioner from inappropriate treatments based on careless assumptions. You may have to see more than one type of practitioner about your problem, for instance a rheumatologist, orthopaedic consultant and a physiotherapist. Even if they are in communication with each other, they will all still ask you for the details of what has happened to your knee. This may seem unnecessary, but each practitioner has a different perspective and needs to ask the questions from a particular point of view.

You can make the process of taking the history more efficient by preparing an accurate written record of the problem to take with you to the consultation. This is especially useful if you are the responsible adult accompanying a child, as children often have difficulty remembering what happened when, and this may be compounded by shyness or fear.

The practitioner will ask you for details of how the problem started, the pain behaviour and how it limits your activities. The questions will vary according to whether you suffered an injury or whether your knee problem started without an obvious external cause. You will also need to reveal background factors relating to your medical history and your lifestyle. All such information is of course strictly confidential between yourself and the practitioner. Every ethically qualified practitioner is obliged to keep accurate records of patient care. In Britain, these must be kept for a minimum of eight years by law, and you have the right to see your medical records should you so choose.

It is in your interest to be truthful. For instance, you may be involved in a legal case for damages relating to your knee problem. Do not be tempted to invent or cover up details of the injury, or to exaggerate your pain and disability in the hope of enhancing your claim. An experienced specialist will always be able to uncover this type of dishonesty, and it is likely to tell against you. It has also been known for patients to pretend that a problem is recent rather than chronic, if their private medical insurance schemes will not cover long-standing problems. If this dishonesty is found out, which it usually is, the insurance company will withhold payment for any treatment, and this can leave the patient with a very large bill, if investigations and surgery have already been performed.

The questions you will be asked by the practitioner will cover aspects of your medical background, your lifestyle, and the knee problem itself. The questions about your knee problem will depend on how it started. If you suffered an injury, the questions are straightforward. If your pain came on without any obvious cause, the questions have to be more searching in order to establish what might have happened.

Questions about your general medical history

- Have you ever suffered from any significant illnesses such as tuberculosis, rheumatic fever or glandular fever?
- When did you last have any notable illness requiring time off school or work, or in bed?
- Do you have any problems with your digestion, such as irritable bowel syndrome?
- Do you have any problems with your urinary system?
- Is there a family history of conditions such as rheumatoid arthritis or heart disease?
- Do you take any medicines for any reason?
- *Females*: Do you take the contraceptive pill or hormone replacement therapy (HRT)?
- Do you have any known allergies?
- Have you had any previous injuries or accidents affecting your legs or back?

Questions about your lifestyle

- Do you take regular exercise or do sport?
- How much physical activity do you do each day and each week?
- Do you normally do fitness training, and if so what kind?
- Had your physical activities been curtailed for any reason before your knee problem started?
- Do you have to sit or stand still for long periods each day (for instance studying or working)?
- Do you drive long distances or for long periods of time?
- Do you eat regular well-balanced meals?
- How much water do you drink every day?
- What is your alcohol consumption (if any)?
- Do you smoke, and if so how much?
- Have you suffered from emotional stress recently?
- Have you felt over-tired for any reason?

What you need to say about an injury

- When did the injury happen?
- What exactly happened? (Did the knee twist, jar, get wrenched or hit?)
- Have you had a similar injury to this knee before?
- What shoes were you wearing and what surface were you on?
- Did you feel pain immediately? If so, exactly where?
- If the pain came on later, how much later? What were you doing at the time?
- Did you feel pain anywhere else apart from the knee?
- Did you notice any swelling? If so, exactly where? Did it appear immediately or only some time after the accident?
- Does the knee give way?
- Does the knee feel stiff?
- Does the knee 'catch', 'pop', click or lock? If so, in what situations?
- How bad is the pain now?
- What brings on the pain?
- How does the pain behave: do you have pain on movement, at rest, sitting, standing, walking, running, hopping, lying in bed, turning over in bed?
- Can the pain be relieved? If so, how?

Questions about knee pain whose cause is unclear

- Does the problem affect one or both knees?
- When did the pain start?
- What exactly were you doing at the time?
- What were you doing immediately before the problem started?
- Had you been doing any unusual activities?
- Had you been ill or felt unwell or unduly fatigued?
- Had you been worried, or under unusual pressure?
- Had you made any changes to your normal diet?
- Is there any pattern to the pain?
- Have you noticed pain in any other joints?
- Is there pain when you are at rest and not doing physical activities?
- Is there pain on any particular movements or activities?
- Do you feel pain at night?
- Do you feel stiffness in the knee(s)?
- Is there noticeable swelling?
- Have you noticed a feeling of heat in the knee(s)?
- Are the symptoms consistent or fluctuating?
- Can you ease the pain? If so, how?

THE PHYSICAL ASSESSMENT

When examining your knee, the practitioner will need to see both your legs, so you should wear shorts or modest underwear. If you do sports, you should bring your sports shoes and any foot orthotics or protective knee supports with you. If you hate having people touch you, you should warn the practitioner at the start of the consultation. If you are nervous about being alone with the practitioner, you should be accompanied by a person of your choice.

The assessment is a physical examination, usually based on seeing and feeling, although the skilled blind practitioner can gain all the information needed through feel alone. Visually, the practitioner can see whether your knees look the same, whether there is swelling, change in skin colour, loss of muscle bulk, and major or minor joint deformity. By touching (technically, palpating) your knees, the practitioner can identify abnormal temperature or temperature differences between the two sides, areas of tenderness, and abnormal muscle tone. To check the joint mobility and how it feels when moved, the practitioner performs passive movements while you keep your muscles relaxed. Guided assisted movements may be done to see how well you can co-ordinate to follow a chosen pattern of movement. By applying pressure to resist movements as you try to perform them, the practitioner can assess the strength, efficiency and co-ordination of the working muscles.

This physical process has to be done with due regard for the patient's pain, and awareness of the patient's possible fears. The practitioner touches the patient gently but firmly, avoiding painful pressure on sensitive tissues. The passive movements for checking joint mobility are not forced to any painful extreme, because the practitioner is guided by signals which warn that the end of the knee's range of movement has been reached and further movement will be painful.

Practitioners use different testing methods according to what they need to know and according to the level of pain and disability in your knee. For instance, the rheumatologist looks for signs of inflammation or infection, the orthopaedic surgeon tests for internal damage or derangement which might warrant an operation, and the physiotherapist assesses functional impairment. How many checks are done and the order in which they are done may vary according to the practitioner and the problem. All practitioners try to establish how much pain you feel in your knee, whether it occurs on any particular movements, and what causes it. They all compare your two knees and both legs.

There are usually several elements to the physical assessment, and your knee will be examined in various positions. Your knee will be assessed while still and in motion. You may be asked to move your knee actively on your own; the practitioner may guide it as you move it; the practitioner may move your knee or your whole leg passively while it is relaxed. Using passive movements, the practitioner can check the overall freedom of the knee and leg, and the more subtle accessory movements which are necessary for the knee's main actions, but which you cannot perform actively at will. Some passive tests involve manipulating the knee in order to check whether torn tissues are blocking the movement or creating laxity in the joint.

If you are able to stand and take weight through your injured leg, part of the assessment may be done with you standing up, the rest with you sitting, or lying down on your back, front or side.

If your knee is grossly swollen or inflamed, the functional assessment process is limited, because movements which might increase the effusion have to be avoided. You will only be asked to do those movements which do not cause pain, usually keeping the knee straight to avoid stressing the joint. You will not be asked to bend the knee under your bodyweight, and the practitioner will not perform manual tests which twist or stretch the knee painfully.

FUNCTIONAL ASSESSMENT TESTS

The purpose of functional testing from the physiotherapist's point of view is to find out what is wrong in order to identify the treatment priorities for successful functional rehabilitation. What the physiotherapist needs to decide is what kind of treatments for pain and swelling are necessary, if any; what the knee's functional deficits are; how the rehabilitation exercise programme should be constructed; and what self-help measures the patient should be advised to use.

When the patient is able to walk and take weight through the injured leg, I normally do the functional tests first with the patient standing, second with the patient lying prone (on the stomach) on the couch, third with the patient lying on his or her back, and finally with the patient sitting up on the couch with his or her legs straight. If the patient is non-weightbearing and using crutches, I place the patient in a comfortable position on the couch straight away and limit the assessment to the minimum.

Functional checks while you are standing up

● As you stand with your knees relaxed, the practitioner compares the contours and skin colour of your knees, and the alignment of your legs and feet. The practitioner looks for swelling, redness or pallor in the knee, any visible imbalance in the leg muscles, distortion of the leg bones, and abnormalities in the position of your feet.

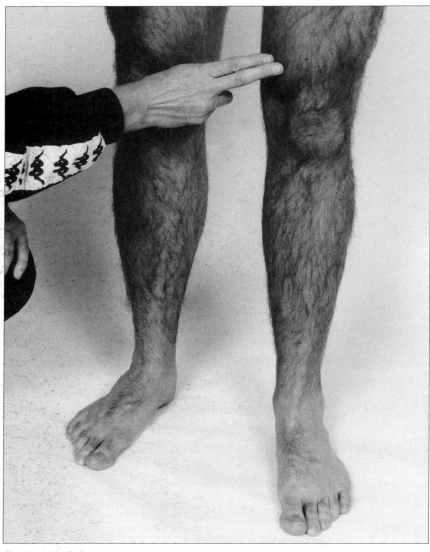

Checking VMO function as it contracts and relaxes in the standing position

- You are asked to tighten your thigh muscles, straightening your knees, then relax them. The practitioner assesses whether your knee-cap is moving awkwardly, and how well you can control the contraction and release of the front-thigh muscles on each side, and asks whether the movement causes any pain.
- You are asked to stand on one leg and hold your balance on each leg

Testing balance mechanisms

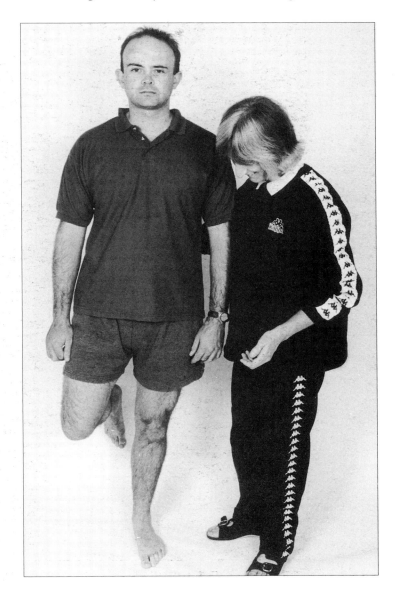

in turn. This tests your static balance mechanisms from the foot and ankle through the whole leg. You are asked if the position causes any pain.

- You are asked to stand on one leg and lift the other out sideways a few times without putting your foot down, on each side in turn. This shows whether you have any weakness or imbalance affecting your

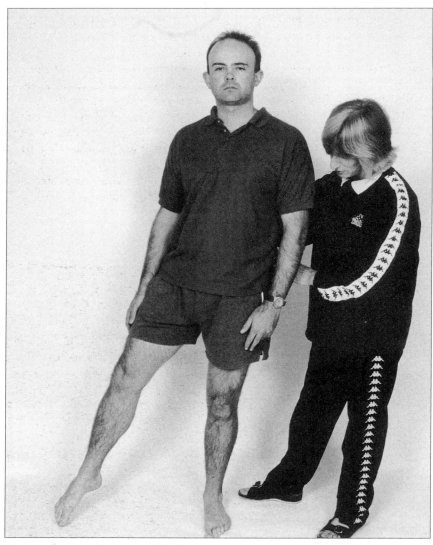

Testing balance mechanisms and hip function

hip on either side. The practitioner watches to see if you lean over sideways as you lift the moving leg, if you have difficulty holding your balance, and if you can perform the movement symmetrically. You are asked if the movement causes any pain in the standing or moving leg.

- You are asked to stand on one leg and go up and down on your toes a few times, keeping your knee absolutely straight, first on one leg, then the other. The practitioner compares the two sides, watching for inability to keep the knee straight, difficulty in going right up on to the toes, difficulty in controlling the reverse movement, and difficulty in holding your balance.

- Standing with your feet slightly apart and parallel, you are asked to go up on to your toes and squat down as fast and as far as you can, keeping your back straight and without putting your heels down. The practitioner watches for asymmetry or difficulty, limitation of movement, or hesitation. You are asked if the movement causes pain.

- Standing with your feet slightly apart and parallel, you are asked to go up on your toes and squat down slowly as far as possible, staying on your toes, then come up again quickly to lock your knees straight. The practitioner checks whether you can do the movement symmetrically and without pain at any point.

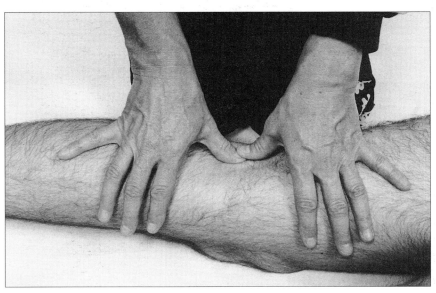

Palpating the back of the knee to test for tightness or tenderness

Tests when you are lying on your stomach

- The practitioner asks whether your kneecap is painful as you lie with it pressing on the surface of the couch. If it is, a support such as a folded towel is placed under your thigh to relieve the pressure.
- The practitioner gently presses the backs of the knees to check whether there is warmth, swelling, or tenderness or tightness in any of the soft tissues, comparing the two knees.
- You are asked to bend your knee as far as you comfortably can and straighten it. The practitioner asks if any part of the movement is painful. The range and quality of the movement are assessed, and note taken if the movement is limited or if you tend to swivel the knee inwards or outwards as you bend it. The practitioner watches

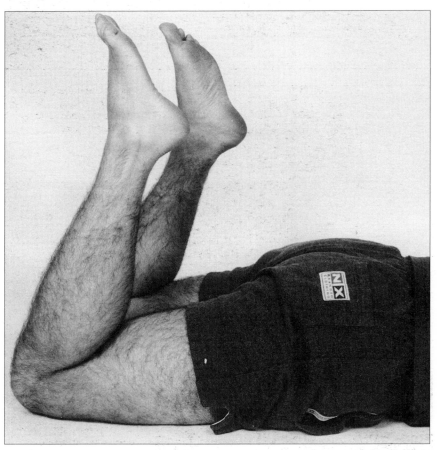

Testing active range of knee flexion, in this case limited on both sides, but more so on the right leg, a sign of overload following a left knee injury

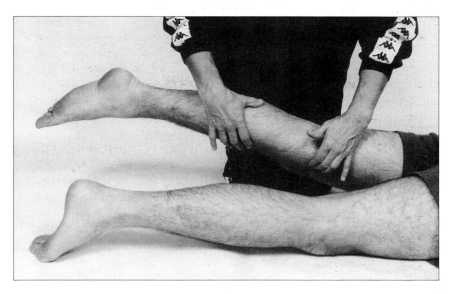

Testing the patient's ability to extend the leg backwards while keeping the knee locked

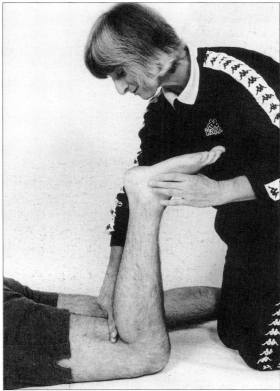

Testing the function of the hamstrings, especially biceps femoris, against gravity and light manual resistance

to see if the hamstring tendons work symmetrically, or if the inner two hamstrings contract more forcefully than the biceps femoris tendon on the outer side of the knee.

- The practitioner carefully bends your knee passively, pressing your foot towards your bottom, while you keep the muscles completely relaxed. The injured knee may be less mobile than the other, but sometimes the front-thigh muscles of the non-injured leg are the tighter, because of overload.
- The practitioner asks you to straighten your knee and lift your leg up a little way behind you, keeping the knee locked straight. You may find it difficult to keep the knee locked straight once it is lifted off the couch, and you may find the movement painful, or harder to do with one leg than the other.
- The practitioner asks you to bend your knee while he or she resists the movement by holding your heel, to test the basic strength and efficiency of the hamstrings. The two sides are compared.
- The practitioner tests the efficiency of your biceps femoris by asking you to bend your knee while keeping your foot turned outwards, away from the other leg, against manual resistance.
- The practitioner asks you to tuck your toes under your feet and straighten both knees. The two sides are compared.

Functional checks as you lie on one side.

- You are asked to lock your uppermost knee straight, and lift the leg upwards away from the other leg. The practitioner notes any pain, or difficulty in keeping the leg in line with the rest of the body. The movement is repeated on the other side.
- Ober's test: the underneath leg is slightly bent, and the practitioner bends your uppermost knee to a right angle, keeping the hip straight (in neutral), and gently allows the upper leg to drop downwards. The amount by which the leg drops behind the lower leg indicates the degree of flexibility in the iliotibial tract. The test is repeated on the other side for comparison.

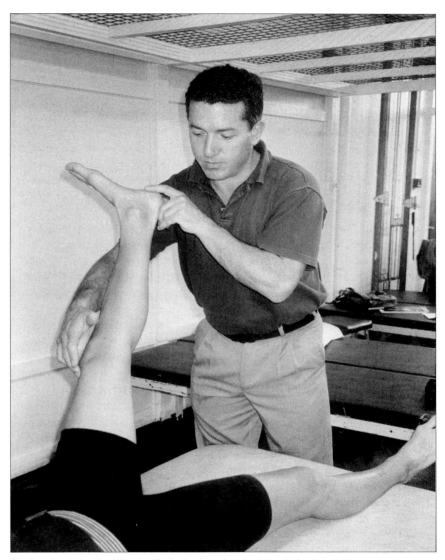

Testing the patient's ability to lift the leg keeping the knee locked straight

Functional tests as you lie on your back

- Lying on your back with your knees straight, you let your legs relax. This shows the angle at which your hips splay. The practitioner notes whether your feet roll outwards to a normal degree, or whether one leg turns out more than the other.

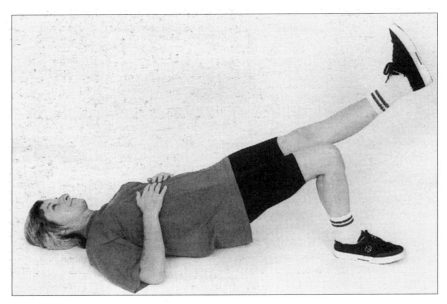

Pelvic lift with one knee straight to test hamstring and back muscle efficiency

- The practitioner bends your knee and hip, then gently presses your leg in an arc from side to side, keeping your hip fully bent. This tests the hip's mobility and sensitivity. The practitioner notes any limitation of movement, pain reactions felt around the hip region or in the groin, and imbalance between the two sides. If the knee is painful when it is held bent, the practitioner exerts the pressure on the back of the thigh just above and behind the knee.
- The practitioner lifts your leg gently upwards, supporting your knee in the straight position, to test the length of your hamstrings and to check for any nerve irritation which might stem from a back problem. The two sides are compared.
- The practitioner asks you to turn your leg outwards, lock your knee straight, and lift your leg straight upwards keeping the knee locked. Failure to maintain the knee extension, called 'extension lag', is noted, and the two sides are compared.
- The practitioner positions you with one knee bent, the other leg held straight upwards so that the knees are level, and you are asked to lift your bottom upwards, maintaining the leg position. This tests the efficiency of the hamstring and lower back muscles on either side.

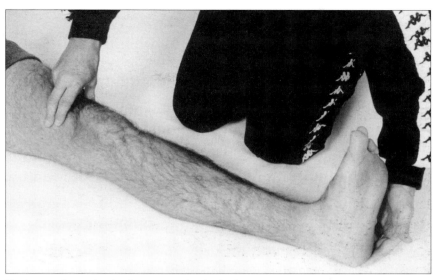

Testing passive and active hyperextension in the knee

Functional tests as you sit with your legs straight in front of you

- The practitioner moves the kneecap gently from side to side and around to check whether it is immobile, tethered down in any part, or unnaturally mobile because of extra fluid around the bone.
- The practitioner asks you to tighten and relax your front-thigh muscles gently, to show whether the kneecap deviates noticeably, and how well you can control the contraction and relaxation of the front-thigh muscles, especially vastus medialis obliquus, on either side.
- The practitioner straightens your knee fully, supporting the foot pointing upwards to check whether your knee is blocked in fixed flexion, has normal extension mobility, hyperextends to a normal degree, or hyperextends abnormally. The two legs are compared.
- The practitioner straightens your knee fully, pulling your heel up to keep your foot pointing upwards, asks you to contract the thigh muscles, then asks you to hold the knee locked straight and lets go of the foot while keeping contact with the vastus medialis obliquus muscle. If the VMO is weak, it feels flabby, the knee cannot hold the locked position, and the foot drops downwards. The two knees are compared.
- You are asked to straighten your knee hard and lift your leg straight upwards as far as you can. Any extension lag is noted, and the two sides are compared.

INVESTIGATIONS

If there is a possibility that you could have an infection, inflammatory condition or some kind of illness, the doctor or surgeon will order blood tests. To establish what internal damage might have happened, the doctor or surgeon will order investigations. X-rays show up bone damage and changes in the alignment of the bones. Arthrograms are special X-rays taken after a positive-contrast material has been injected into the knee, and they are especially useful for showing up injuries in the semilunar cartilages and problems in the articular cartilage. Computerized tomography, known as CT scanning, is a technique which translates a series of X-ray views taken across the knee into a three-dimensional picture of the joint. It can reveal injuries to the soft tissues including cruciate ligament tears, bone problems including fractures and tumours, and subtle distortions of the joint alignment, especially in the kneecap (patellofemoral) joint. Magnetic resonance imaging (MRI) uses the interaction of magnetic and electromagnetic fields with the knee's tissues to create a visual image of the joint. It can show up damage to the bones, articular cartilage and soft tissues inside the knee. Less often used for the diagnosis of knee problems is ultrasonography, as it does not give as much information as other forms of investigation, although it can identify clearly problems like Baker's cysts and injuries to the patellar tendon.

All the modern techniques of investigating the body systems are constantly changing according to the apparently never-ending improvements in technology. The choice of investigations depends on the nature of the patient's problem, and sometimes on the availability of the apparatus. Investigations are always kept to the minimum necessary, especially when the patient is a child, because the process can be stressful, and over-exposure to X-rays, for instance, can be harmful. Most of the sophisticated investigative techniques show a wide range of problems very accurately, but none is absolutely foolproof. Surgeons still often find unexpected damage when they operate and actually look inside the knee through the arthroscope.

Surgery and conservative treatments

9

Physical treatments cannot mend torn knee structures. In some cases the torn tissues around the knee heal naturally after being wholly or partially torn, but the internal structures like the semilunar cartilages and the cruciate ligaments do not repair themselves. If it is likely that the knee has suffered internal damage, the orthopaedic surgeon may be called upon by the general practitioner to diagnose the injury, and to decide whether the damage warrants surgery.

An operation is required only when there is obvious disruption to the knee's structures which is impeding proper function. This can be caused by injury, or sometimes by diseases, such as rheumatoid arthritis. If an operation is not considered necessary or desirable, at least in the first instance, the surgeon may choose to perform other techniques. Removing excess fluid (aspiration) from the knee may be necessary, to relieve the pressure on the joint, prevent damage to the articular surfaces, and to analyse the fluid in case it reveals inflammation or infection. Occasionally, the surgeon will inject the knee: this may be done, for instance, to relieve localized pain in one of the more superficial structures, such as the medial or lateral ligament. Injecting the knee joint itself, or any of the major tendons, is usually avoided, because of the risk of causing damage. Manipulation under anaesthetic is another treatment which is used in the rare cases when knee movement is completely blocked, and all other methods of releasing it have failed.

IF YOU NEED AN OPERATION

Many types of knee injuries and problems require surgery. Some operations have to be performed as emergencies, so you have little choice about whether to have the operation or not.

In many cases, the need for surgery shows up at a later stage, when the knee fails to recover fully from an injury and impedes your normal activities whether at home, school, college, work, sport or leisure. Later-stage surgery, which is called elective surgery, puts you in the position of having to choose whether you really want to go through with it. You have the right to refuse. You may be frightened by the idea of an operation. You may wonder whether it is really necessary, or the best option available. You may be confused about which surgeon to see and which operation you might need or be offered. It may be inconvenient to have to commit time to the operation and recovery in the context of your studies, work or social commitments.

On the other hand, the idea of having an operation might seem to offer a beguilingly simple solution to your knee problem: you go to sleep, the surgeon sets to work, you wake up and all is well. In fact, you have to be prepared to work towards your functional recovery by doing remedial exercises before and after the operation. Any knee operation, however minor, represents further trauma to an already weakened joint. Concentrated effort is needed before and afterwards for a full recovery.

WHAT YOU NEED TO KNOW ABOUT ANY PROPOSED OPERATION

Once the surgeon says that an operation is needed for your knee problem, you need to ask some relevant questions. Don't be afraid to ask any questions that are on your mind. The surgeon may seem short of time, and may not be forthcoming with explanations. You have to understand that he is busy making efficient clinical decisions, and may not be aware of your individual worries. As the surgeon has a duty to explain the nature and consequences of the surgical procedure he is proposing to perform on you, it is up to you to ask for more detailed clarification if there is any particular aspect you don't understand. It is especially important to establish clearly what is involved in proposed surgery for a child or teenager, so parents should always be prepared to persist with relevant questions until they are confident they can make an appropriate decision about the operation on the child's behalf.

It can be helpful to write down in advance the questions you want to ask, so that you can run through them without hesitation, and perhaps note down the answers. If you find that you still have unanswered questions after your consultation with the surgeon, you can write to him expressing your concerns. Try to be as brief and concise as possible, and set out concrete questions for the surgeon to answer.

You may not need or wish to ask all of the following questions, but you can choose those which seem pertinent to your situation.

Questions about the operation

- What exactly does the proposed operation entail?
- Is the operation urgent?
- Can I, or should I, wait to see if the problem gets better with rehabilitation treatment before making a decision about going ahead with surgery?
- Is it possible to return to strenuous sports following this operation?
- Is it possible to return to strenuous sports if I don't have the operation?
- Are there any possible complications of the operation: if so, what are they?
- How long will I have to wait before I have the operation?
- What should I be doing to prepare myself for the operation?
- If there is a long delay, what should I be doing to help the knee in the meanwhile?
- Can I have physiotherapy treatment in the period before the operation?

Questions about recovering from the operation

- How mobile will I be immediately after the operation?
- How long will I have to stay in hospital?
- Will I have to use crutches after the operation, and if so, for how long?
- What kind of a scar will I have?
- Will the knee be swollen after the operation?
- Will the knee be painful post-operatively?
- How soon will I be able to take a shower or bath?
- Will I have physiotherapy treatment?
- How soon can I drive a car, or ride a bicycle or motorcycle after the operation?
- How quickly can I return to school, college or work?
- How quickly will I be able to return to sport?

ESTABLISHING CONFIDENCE IN YOUR SURGEON

It is very important for you to be sure that the operation the surgeon is proposing to do is essential. You must have complete confidence in the surgeon. Remember that any form of operation, even so-called 'keyhole'

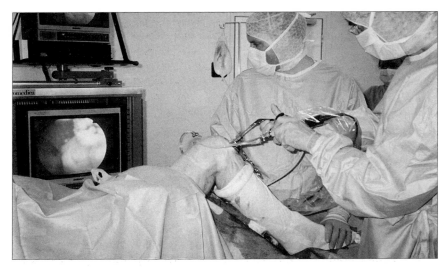

Sophisticated modern surgical techniques have made knee operations safer and more accurate. The camera attached to the arthroscope allows the surgeon an enlarged view of the inside of the knee

surgery (arthroscopy) represents trauma to the knee, so it should not be undertaken lightly, by either the surgeon or yourself. If you have doubts or worries about the surgeon or the operation you should express them to your general practitioner.

The surgeon's main role is to decide on whether an operation is necessary, if so, which operation, and whether he is the competent person to perform it. If possible, your operation should be done by a senior or consultant surgeon who specializes in knee problems, rather than a trainee or junior. If you have a complex problem, and the surgeon does not have the expertise needed to deal with it, he should be honest enough to admit it, and to refer you to a more specialized surgeon.

You need to know that your surgeon is competent, and confident of success. In the case of children, the surgeon must be specialized in dealing with young people during their growth and development phases. As in any other branch of medicine, new procedures for treating different conditions are being developed all the time. If the proposed operation for your knee problem is new, you need to know how well established it is, why the surgeon has chosen that particular procedure, and how certain he is that the operation will be succeed. Most surgeons monitor their patients after surgery: sometimes over several years following complicated operations. If the surgeon recommends physiotherapy treatment after the operation, this is another guarantee that you will be monitored over a period of time.

Surgeons vary in their attitudes to their patients. While some are charming and genuinely or apparently caring, others can seem offhand, brusque, rude or unfeeling. It is hard to have confidence in a surgeon who has failed to make you feel at ease; harder still if he has been offhand with you. However, your priority is to establish whether he is competent to do the required operation for you, and whether he is the best person available. Personality differences should be seen as unimportant.

Questions for confidence

- How long has the proposed operation been used by orthopaedic surgeons?
- How many of these operations have you performed?
- Will you do the operation on my knee yourself?
- Will you follow up my case and monitor my recovery after the operation?
- Do you recommend that your patients have physiotherapy treatment after the operation?
- What percentage of your patients have returned to full physical activities following this operation?
- Have you treated many cases which have failed to reach full recovery?
- Do any of your patients develop infections or other complications: if so, what percentage?

SEEKING A SECOND OPINION

If you are totally dissatisfied with what your surgeon has told you about your knee problem and his proposed solution, it is sensible to seek a second opinion, and it is your right to do so. Sometimes it is worth consulting a second surgeon simply for reassurance that the first surgeon's diagnosis and proposed treatment are reasonably based and likely to succeed. The fact that you have received a second opinion does not prevent you from proceeding with treatment from the original surgeon.

The correct ethical way to go about obtaining a second opinion is to be referred to the second surgeon by your general practitioner. You may have identified the surgeon of your choice through private research or recommendation, but your general practitioner acts as the central reference point. The general practitioner maintains a record of all the test results and opinions about your problem, so that any further practitioners dealing with you can be informed of the relevant facts.

Seek a second opinion

- if you wish to double-check that the diagnosis is likely to be correct and the proposed treatment regime is appropriate
- if you lack confidence in your surgeon
- if you are not sure that the proposed procedure is the right one for your problem

Avoid surgery

- if you know you react badly to a general anaesthetic
- if you are too frightened by the idea of an operation to cope
- if you feel your surgeon might not be competent to perform a successful operation
- if you are likely to be operated on by a trainee or junior surgeon without supervision by a senior
- if you do not know who will perform the operation
- if there is any doubt about the nature of your knee problem
- if more than one surgeon is unsure about the need for an operation
- if more than one surgeon feels that no operation can help your problem
- if your knee problem is getting better with rehabilitation treatment

DIFFICULTIES IN RECOVERY AFTER AN OPERATION

Rehabilitation treatment is needed after surgery, as there is always a certain amount of muscle inhibition and functional loss, even after the most minor operation. However, some surgeons think rehabilitation is not necessary and the operation is sufficient to restore function. A few think that rehabilitation treatment will spoil the good effects of the operation. The patient is therefore encouraged to do 'normal activities', and then progress to more physically demanding tasks or sports as desired.

The results of this approach can be less than satisfactory. Very often recovery is not achieved, so the patient has to attend for rehabilitation treatment at a late stage. As the patient has usually been led to believe that full recovery would be achieved by this time, it can be very frustrating to learn that the rehabilitation process is only just beginning. If the patient has done too much too soon while left to his or her own devices, new problems may have been created in the operated knee which may even need further surgical repair. Even if full recovery does seem to have happened and the patient manages to return to full activities, there is always a risk that if the patient has been left with even the most tiny functional deficit, there will be muscle and joint imbalance which may well lead to degenerative change (osteoarthritis) in the operated knee, the other knee or either hip.

Another problem which can arise if the patient does not receive rehabilitation treatment post-operatively is pain after the anaesthetic effects of the operation have worn off. Sometimes, the pain feels very similar to the pain from before the operation. This naturally makes the patient worry that the operation has failed. This anxiety can be spared if a competent practitioner is monitoring the knee and can work out why it is painful and what needs to be done. In fact, the pain can be a reaction to the trauma of the operation, or due to excessive strain on the knee before it is ready, or linked to habitually poor postural and movement patterns caused by the knee's functional deficits. Most often, post-operative pain is resolved by appropriate treatment and rehabilitation measures.

CONSERVATIVE TREATMENT FOR PAIN AND SWELLING

Conservative treatment means not having an operation. Treatments are not standardized. For one thing, treatment methods are constantly changing and developing. For another, for any given problem there are often several ways of effecting a cure, or at least improving the situation. Practitioners develop their own individual systems for dealing with injuries and pain syndromes, and they do not always agree with each other about treatment and rehabilitation methods. There is no single prescription which is guaranteed to cure the various sorts of knee problems in different patients. Physical treatment systems have to be flexible to a certain extent, to allow for individual differences between patients and their responses to the treatment process. Every method which achieves its desired goals is appropriate and right.

Physical treatments for pain and swelling

Physical treatments are those which are applied externally. Ice and contrast hot-and-cold applications are among the simplest ways of relieving pain and swelling in most knee problems. Physiotherapists and sometimes other practitioners may use electrotherapy machines, very often interferential therapy, transcutaneous electronic nerve stimulation (TENS), laser and ultrasound. Manual therapy, shiatsu and aromatherapy can all be beneficial for reducing or curing the symptoms.

Following any knee injury or after surgery I use gentle massage and soft-tissue manipulation, sometimes combined with diadynamic therapy to reduce swelling and pain. Diadynamic therapy uses low-frequency electrical currents with an element of direct current to create chemical changes in the tissues between the two electrodes, which are placed on either side of the knee or above and below it. The effect of the currents is to improve absorption of the excess fluid in the swollen knee. It cannot be used if metal has been implanted or if there is a circulatory problem such as a blood clot in the knee; otherwise it is considered a very safe technique.

If a painful knee is hot and swollen because of inflammation through disease or food intolerance, it will be very sensitive, so electrotherapy or any invasive treatments will make it much more painful. In this case, I treat the swelling and pain with very gentle massage which the patient can hardly feel, using fine soft-tissue handling techniques like those developed for the specialized treatment of lymphatic drainage.

Treatments for correcting functional deficits in the knee

Dealing with pain and swelling is the prerequisite for regaining normal function in the injured joint.

Joint movement limitation may be treated with manual therapy techniques, gentle manipulation and mobilizing techniques. Any forceful pain-causing manoeuvres are avoided because they are likely to increase pain, swelling and inhibition in the joint. The practitioner may increase joint mobility by bending and straightening the knee gently and rhythmically through its available range, or by holding it bent or straight at its limit to stretch the muscles passively. In most cases of joint limitation the practitioner has to mobilize the knee's accessory movements by holding the joint bent to 90 degrees and twisting it gently. Sometimes the tibiofibular joint has to be freed by gentle manipulation of the head of the fibula against the shin-bone.

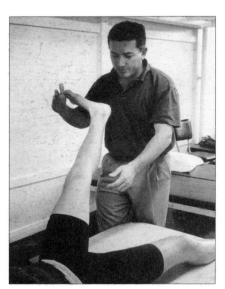

Neuromuscular energizing therapy techniques for the VMO and related muscles

Weakened or inhibited muscles can be helped with electrical muscle stimulation (see p.147), or facilitation techniques, which are movements guided by the therapist. Proprioceptive neuromuscular facilitation (PNF) is the traditional technique for reviving co-ordination through patterns of movement performed by the

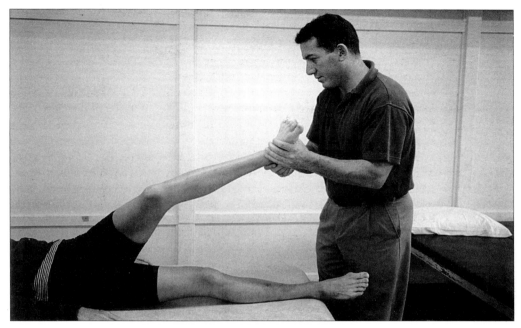

Neuromuscular energizing therapy techniques for the hip abductors and outer thigh muscles

patient against the manual resistance provided by the therapist. Neuromuscular energizing therapy (NET) is a modern system of facilitation. With NET, the therapist uses very light manual guidance through patterns of movement to revive co-ordination of muscle groups and stimulate the patient's nervous system and internal energy to appropriate levels for normal activity.

Feedback and guidance are important for teaching you correct movements, so that you can then benefit from the accurate remedial exercises which are the core of the self-help recovery programme.

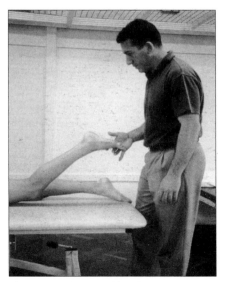

Neuromuscular energizing therapy techniques for the hamstrings

Pain-relieving and anti-inflammatory drugs

For immediate relief of pain you can take non-prescription painkillers, or drugs may be prescribed by your doctor. These may be painkillers or non-steroidal anti-inflammatory drugs (NSAIDs), which are designed to help the healing processes. Sometimes a combination of drugs is given. Any drugs prescribed by the doctor or surgeon must be taken as directed, especially as some may have a bad effect on the stomach if taken wrongly. If you react badly to a prescribed drug, you should tell the practitioner immediately. If you do not want to take oral medicines for any reason, you should make that clear before they are prescribed.

The pain relief afforded by drugs does not mean that your problem is instantly cured. You must be careful not to fall into the trap of assuming that you can go back to normal activities which stress your knee, just because you cannot feel the pain in it any longer. The drugs are a temporary measure to make your painful knee more comfortable. The fact that you need them is a warning that your knee is not ready for normal action yet, so you must be patient and wait until your knee is painfree without the help of drugs before you stress the joint.

If you are prescribed drugs, make sure you keep them out of reach of children and pets. Never pass them on to other people. If you have any left over, take them back to the pharmacist for safe disposal. The same guidelines apply to homoeopathic medicines as to pharmaceutical drugs. You must beware of the temptation to think that any medicine can be a self-administered magic cure, bought 'off the shelf'. Homoeopathy, medicines and the human body are complicated, and it is all too easy to make a mistake with self-help medication.

TREATMENT FOR CHRONIC PAIN

Long-standing pain following an injury or operation is always a difficult symptom for the practitioner to deal with. It should never be ignored, even if the patient seems to be complaining unduly. It can sometimes be tempting to dismiss a complaint of pain as 'psychological' or 'all in the mind', but this will not help the patient. When the practitioner does not take complaints of pain seriously, the patient quickly loses faith in the practitioner's judgement and level of care.

In most common knee problems, resolving the pain depends on accurate assessment and appropriate treatment. If pain persists despite initial treatment, it can mean that the original diagnosis was mistaken or incomplete, that compensatory mechanisms have added to the original pain, or that there is a secondary problem underlying the main one. There may be a need for more detailed investigations and a change of treatment strategy.

If you are anxious, afraid, stressed or depressed, your knee problem will be harder to cure and the pain will be more persistent. Your mind – and particularly your perception of pain – can influence the healing processes. In some cases, emotional disturbances prolong the symptoms of a mechanical knee problem. In rarer cases, the knee symptoms are actually caused by emotional problems.

Dealing with chronic pain requires a flexible and sensitive treatment programme. Remedial exercises are a must, but only within the patient's capacity and within pain limits. Apart from appropriate drug therapy, electrotherapy techniques, especially TENS, can relieve pain. Pain-relieving injections may be tried, usually to the outer structures of the knee only, avoiding the knee joint itself. In some cases, the knee will be protected in a supportive bandage or even a plaster cast, and the patient may have to use crutches to avoid overloading the knee. Wherever possible, total immobilization of the knee is avoided because this can cause even more problems by weakening the muscles and disturbing the blood flow.

Positive thinking is an important part of the cure, and if you find this difficult to achieve, you should seek help from an appropriate practitioner, such as a psychotherapist, clinical psychologist, counsellor or, for more severe illness, psychiatrist.

TREATMENT FOR PSYCHOSOMATIC PAIN

If it is established beyond doubt that the patient is not suffering from any injury, infection, inflammatory process or disease which might explain his or her pain, the patient should be directed through the general practitioner or consultant specialist towards an appropriate practitioner, whether psychotherapist, clinical psychologist or psychiatrist, for treatment according to the nature of the disorder.

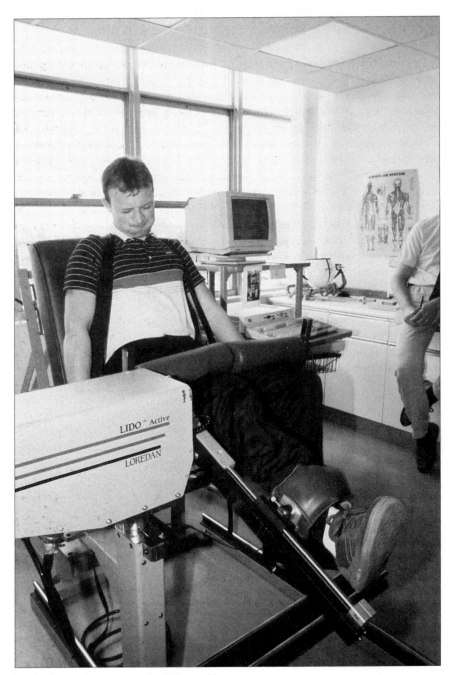

Isokinetic muscle testing on the Lido machine

HOW DO YOU KNOW IF TREATMENT IS WORKING?

When treatment is successful, your knee pain and swelling are reduced, your knee movements become freer, your knee gradually feels more normal, and you should be able progressively to perform the activities of your choice. In the normal way, you know you are getting better because you feel better. Occasionally, fear clouds your perception of your improvement, and you may think you are not getting better when in fact you are. In this situation, it helps if you have objective measurements to judge by, such as the angle to which you can bend your knee, or muscle measurements on testing equipment like the Lido, Kin Com or Cybex.

Sometimes progress is slow, sometimes there are setbacks. If you experience continuing or new problems in your knee you need to try to identify the cause. If you are doing too much or over-stressing the knee through careless posture, you should modify your activities and correct your posture. If your diet is inadequate and you are getting intermittent food intolerance reactions (see p.46), you should monitor and correct this aspect.

Even if you experience temporary setbacks for identifiable reasons, you should notice perceptible improvements week by week, if not day by day. However, if you cannot see any objective signs of your knee problem gradually getting better, the treatment strategy needs to be reviewed.

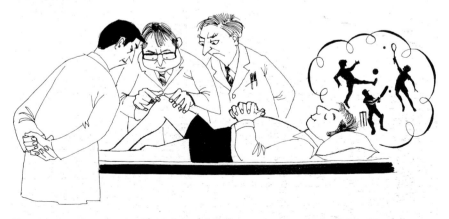

Dreaming won't make your knee better. Passive treatments must be followed by active rehabilitation

WHAT IF THE PROBLEM FAILS TO GET BETTER?

Whether or not you are having treatment, you must take action if your problem is not improving. If the diagnosis was mistaken or not properly established, you may need to have more checks and investigations. If you have not been having ongoing treatment, you should refer to your general practitioner or specialist for further help, or seek a second opinion through your general practitioner if you fail to get satisfaction. If you are under treatment, you should discuss your lack of progress with your practitioner and ask for an explanation and guidance. If you have been given remedial exercises to do at home, you should go through them with your practitioner or another appropriately qualified therapist, in case you are doing them incorrectly or they are no longer appropriate.

If the treatment and advice given are obviously not working, the programme should be changed or discontinued, unless there is a reasonable justification for continuing it. If you lose confidence in the practitioner, ask your general practitioner to refer you to someone else.

Rehabilitation and functional recovery

10

REHABILITATION TREATMENT

Conservative treatment should not mean 'rest, do nothing at all, wait and see', except when there is acute inflammation, which is usually related to an infection or a disease. Treatment should not be limited to pain-relieving techniques alone. A troublesome knee cannot be pronounced fit just because it no longer hurts.

Recovery does not just happen by itself. Rehabilitation is the process through which you recover stability, movement and co-ordination in the knee and its related muscles and joints, and eliminate compensatory mechanisms, in order to do normal activities, including work, sport and leisure. A comprehensive exercise programme includes exercises for the rest of the body and, when appropriate, cardiorespiratory fitness training as well.

In the immediate aftermath of a traumatic injury, damage limitation is needed. The more you can do to preserve the muscles around the knee, the better for your overall recovery. Remedial exercises should start at the earliest stage possible to help the circulation and maintain the leg muscles, and they should be done at regular intervals throughout each day.

An adequate progressive rehabilitation programme can only be set by a practitioner who knows about the structure and functions of the knee, knee problems and exercise therapy. Even if you know a lot about sports and physical training, you will not be able to work out accurately the details of a remedial programme suitable for a particular problem. A qualified therapist can guide you safely through the phases of recovery or improvement, advise on which activities are suitable at any stage, and recommend when you can return to physically demanding activities. If

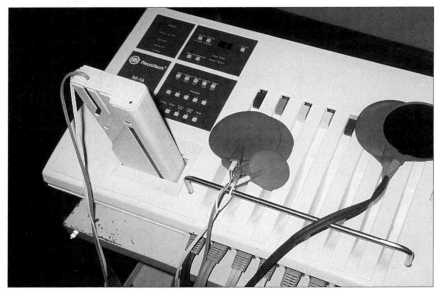

A programmable electrical muscle stimulator with portable mini-stimulator for home use

any problems arise in the course of the treatment programme, the therapist can take or recommend appropriate action.

You must make time every day for your rehabilitation programme, and you must be patient. Rehabilitation is not done to a timescale but according to the responses and capacities of the individual patient. If there are any complications, whether physical or psychological, recovery is slower.

Once the physiotherapist has set out your remedial exercise regime, it is down to you to do the exercises sufficiently and well, as your physiotherapist cannot be with you all the time. Accuracy is essential. The exercises require concentration. Even a few repetitions done well are a worthwhile contribution towards functional recovery, whereas hundreds of exercises done badly are at best a waste of time and at worst may hinder recovery or even cause damage.

Exercise one leg at a time at first, even if you have problems in both knees. Don't try to perform the maximum number of repetitions in the minimum possible time. Don't try too hard. 'Going for the burn' is counterproductive. 'No pain, no gain' is a maxim wholly out of place in the rehabilitation context. If there is pain, there is also inhibition of muscle action, leading to compensatory mechanisms being brought into play to achieve a desired movement.

RECOVERY OF VASTUS MEDIALIS OBLIQUUS: A PRIORITY

The vastus medialis obliquus muscle (VMO) is the quickest of the knee muscles to become dysfunctional through pain and injury, but the slowest to recover, and the most difficult to rehabilitate. Full VMO efficiency is essential for complete recovery from any knee problem.

The VMO has a unique and difficult role in stabilizing the kneecap and locking the knee into full extension. Once it has been weakened, it is very hard to re-train the VMO's controlling nerve mechanisms and co-ordination patterns through exercises alone. Most exercises involving the knee make use of several thigh muscles together. If the VMO is not functioning normally, it cannot benefit from the training effect of the exercises to the same degree as its surrounding muscles. The imbalance between the VMO and the other thigh muscles worsens as a result. This applies especially to straight-leg-raising in the sitting or lying positions.

Traditionally, the straight-leg-raise exercise has been used as the primary exercise in knee rehabilitation, especially after many knee operations, including cartilage removal (meniscectomy). In some hospitals, the ability to perform the straight-leg-raise is the criterion for allowing the patient to go home. However, in the early phases of recovery from an injury or surgical procedure the patient almost invariably cannot lock the knee straight. Doing the exercise with the knee slightly bent (called the extension lag) defeats the purpose of the exercise. Good control of the VMO must be regained before the straight-leg-raise is attempted.

Electrical neuromuscular stimulation is probably the most efficient method of reviving VMO function.

ELECTRICAL NEUROMUSCULAR (MUSCLE) STIMULATION

Electrical neuromuscular or muscle stimulation uses a low-frequency alternating current to activate the motor nerve which controls the target muscle, and so makes the muscle contract. This is not a passive exercise but a re-education technique. The electricity provides an accurate guiding signal which helps the nerve and muscle to respond accurately and efficiently, and the patient has to activate the muscle in conjunction with the current to achieve the training effect.

This technique of muscle re-education is not new. It has been used with success for very many years. It can be done with simple faradic machines, and even with the small muscle-stimulating devices which are sold as 'slimming aids'.

A modern variable muscle stimulator makes it possible to use appropriate frequencies for faster-twitch or slow-twitch muscles. The intensity readout gives the practitioner information about the efficiency of the target muscle, and helps the continuity of treatment from session to session. One ingenious development is the computerized muscle stimulator with a baby stimulator which can be programmed from it for home use. The baby machine also has a 'truth check' device which records exactly how long the patient has used the machine – a powerful motivator to patient compliance with the self-help programme.

For re-education work using a variable muscle stimulator, the pulse rate is usually set at 40 or 50 hertz, pulse width about 50 (for comfort), contraction time 4 seconds, rest phase between contractions 12 seconds. The relatively long relaxation phase is important, as it helps the patient to re-learn how to release the muscle. Once the electrodes have been sited, the current intensity is gradually turned up until there is a slight contraction in the muscle. The more inhibited the target muscle, the higher the intensity needed to make it contract, especially if the patient has a lot of adipose tissue, when the intensity required may be as high as 120 milliamperes. More often, the starting intensity is in the region of 80–90 milliamperes. The current should be the minimum necessary to achieve muscle contraction. It is not the case that 'the stronger the current, the better'. If the current gives a strong sensation, it is harder for the patient to contract the target muscle.

Electrical muscle stimulation for the vastus medialis obliquus

For the vastus medialis obliquus there can be four elements to the muscle work done with the muscle stimulator, although good function is often obtained by using the first two alone.

First, the patient works at fine control, to regain the ability to twitch the muscle and make the kneecap move just a little, without activating the outer quadriceps muscles or the iliotibial band. Second, the patient does full knee-straightening (hyperextension) movements, pressing the knee downwards to lock it and turning the foot to point the toes upwards (in dorsiflexion). Pointing the foot upwards helps give an active stretch to the gastrocnemius muscle, whose tendons are attached behind the knee. The leg may be in the neutral position for this, or turned outwards. For the third element, a small support, such as a rolled-up towel, is placed under the patient's heel, to provide leverage as the patient presses the knee downwards to straighten it. For the fourth, a wedge or roll is placed under the knee, and the knee is straightened from the slightly bent position.

Sometimes contracting the front-thigh muscles causes pain over the front of the knee, especially along the inner side of the kneecap or the pes anserinus. Rubbing ice over the sore area can relieve this, so that the exercise can safely be continued. If it does not, the muscle activity is restricted to the mild twitching movement only, until the more forceful contraction can be achieved without pain.

As the nerve to the VMO becomes more efficient, less intensity is needed to make the muscle contract. The current must feel comfortable at all times and the patient must feel confident, otherwise it will be impossible for the patient to concentrate well enough to make the muscles work accurately. If the patient is extremely nervous of electricity I keep the current to a low level, just enough to give a mild sensation of tingling, until the patient has gained enough confidence to allow the current to be turned up to contraction level.

When electrical muscle stimulation cannot be used

There are very few situations in which the use of electrical muscle stimulation for the VMO is contraindicated. As with other forms of electrotherapy, muscle stimulation is not normally used on patients with pacemakers, or those who have active infections or disease.

In extremely rare cases the patient is too frightened to tolerate the idea of an electric current through the muscle. For these patients, I sometimes

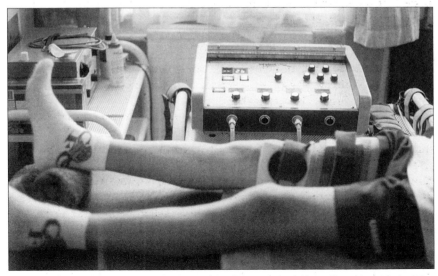

Electrical muscle stimulation for vastus medialis obliquus: with the heel supported, the patient presses the knee downwards to straighten it fully

use biofeedback to heighten their awareness of the VMO function, as this machine does not create a sensation of electricity. Working in front of a mirror to regain VMO control in the standing position is a useful self-help feedback technique. In all cases where muscle stimulation cannot be applied, I use manual therapy techniques, especially those of neuromuscular energizing therapy (NET) (see p.139), to help regain co-ordination between the VMO and its surrounding muscles.

Electrical muscle stimulation for other knee muscles

In some situations, electrical neuromuscular stimulation is used for other muscles around the knee, apart from the VMO.

At the back of the knee, the outer tendon of the hamstring muscles, the biceps femoris, has an important role in stabilizing the knee, especially when the anterior cruciate ligament is defective. For biceps femoris muscle re-education, electrical stimulation can be applied to it when the patient's knee is bent and the foot turned slightly outwards. The patient may sit on a chair and press the heel back against the chair-leg as the current surges. Or the stimulation is done with the patient lying prone (on the stomach), bending the knee while keeping the foot turned outwards. The muscle work may be isometric, when the leg works against a fixed resistance, or dynamic, if the patient bends the knee with a weight attached to his or her foot or ankle, or if the practitioner applies resistance while allowing the knee to bend.

TYPES OF EXERCISES USED FOR KNEE REHABILITATION

Isometric or static exercises

Isometric or static muscle work involves tensing a muscle group without creating movement in the joint which it controls. It is important for maintaining muscle tone in situations where a joint is immobilized, so it is a type of exercise which can and should be done immediately after a knee injury or operation, especially when the leg is encased in bandaging or a plaster cast, unless it causes notable pain.

Any muscle group can work isometrically in any part of its movement range. Although you can contract the front-thigh muscles isometrically with the knee bent by pressing the lower leg against a fixed resistance or doing the 'wall-sit' exercise, it is not to be recommended because it can cause kneecap pain (see Chapter 5). The front-thigh muscles are usually worked isometrically with the knee straight. The so-called 'static quadriceps regime' is a traditional feature of early-stage remedial exercises for knee problems. In this programme, the knee is locked straight, to set the front-thigh muscles isometrically, and the leg is lifted in different directions. In order to involve the hamstrings, gluteals and hip adductors, these exercises are done not only in the sitting or lying positions but also lying on the side and on the stomach.

Isometric front-thigh contractions should be done in the first stage of recovery, and maintained through the subsequent stages in a knee rehabilitation programme. Isometric contractions are usually held for a count of two or slightly more. It is extremely important to relax the muscles completely, for at least a count of five, in between repetitions, in order to let the blood flow through them again. Failure to do this can cause muscle cramp, and may even lead to raised blood pressure.

Isotonic (dynamic) exercises

Isotonic or dynamic exercises involve active joint movement and different kinds of muscle work. Gravity and loading influence the type of muscle work involved in any given movement. When a muscle works against gravity and moves a joint by shortening, the muscle work is concentric. To control the reverse movement the muscles have to pay out eccentrically. Eccentric muscle action is often inefficient in unfit people, or in sports players who have not followed a properly balanced training programme. It is easily undermined by muscle or joint injury, and is harder to recover than concentric action.

Movements and exercises can be defined as weightbearing, partial-weightbearing or non-weightbearing, according to whether the limb is supporting all, some or none of your bodyweight. In modern parlance, open kinetic chain exercises are those in which

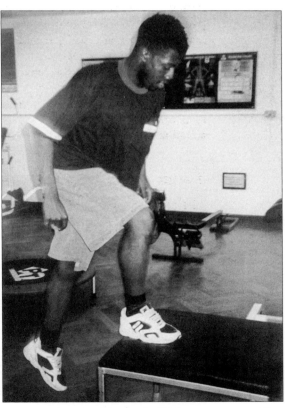

Weightbearing dynamic exercises like step-ups are used in the later stages of rehabilitation for co-ordination, strength and fitness training

the end part of a series of joints is not fixed, while in closed kinetic chain exercises the last joint is stabilized. Non-weightbearing knee exercises are therefore defined as open kinetic chain training, while full and partial weightbearing movements are closed kinetic chain.

When the leg is weightbearing, it receives a lot of sensory information through the nerves in the sole of the foot and the other weightbearing joints, the foot, ankle and hip, so that in closed kinetic chain exercises it can be harder for the patient to isolate the VMO function and to avoid compensatory mechanisms. However, weightbearing through the foot is important for promoting the circulatory flow through the leg, so some standing exercises are usually introduced as quickly as possible to the programme.

Progressive resistance exercises (PRE) are used to build up muscle strength. Free weights such as dumb-bells, barbells, weights boots and strap-on weights can be used for non-weightbearing and weightbearing exercises against gravity. Pulley systems, clinibands or bicycle inner tubes allow for more complex movements with light loading. Fixed-weights machines such as the Nautilus, Powersport, David and Norsk systems make weight training easier and safer by providing stable starting positions for each movement.

Strengthening exercises involving increasing knee movement are

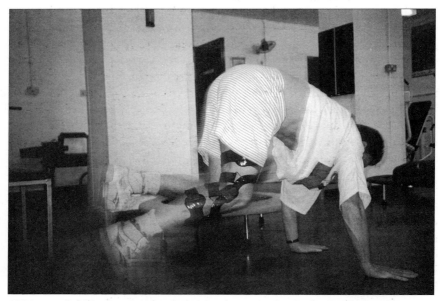

Alternate leg thrusts can be used as early-stage plyometric exercises for fitness and co-ordination

usually the second stage of recovery in most knee problems. All the knee's muscle groups are strengthened, to create good muscle balance. The selection of exercises is guided by any pain reactions. For instance, leg press machine exercises pushing against a load with the feet to straighten the knee from the bent position, start with only a small range of movement, which gradually increases. Knee extension exercises, straightening the knee by bringing the foot upwards with a weight over the ankle or foot, are usually only possible at a later stage because of the traction effect on the main knee joint. Eccentric muscle action should always be emphasized.

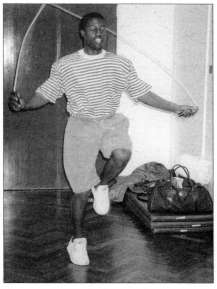

Plyometric exercises like skipping (rope-jumping) are used in the very last stages of rehabilitation leading into full sports participation

Weightbearing strengthening and co-ordination exercises such as quarter-squats, half-squats and full-squats are gradually introduced into the programme from about the third phase of recovery, once the knee has recovered a good range of movement and reasonable strength in the non-weightbearing weight-resisted exercises. Confidence is often a problem. It is usually easier to do weightbearing knee-bending movements quickly at first, progressing to the slower movements which are more demanding of eccentric muscle control.

Full squatting may not be possible in certain situations, such as after total knee replacement surgery. Wherever possible, the ability to squat fully should be recovered: the movement provides lubrication inside the whole knee, prevents excessive weightbearing pressure on limited areas of the joint surfaces, and is also important for lifting objects from the floor safely without straining your back.

Plyometrics

Plyometrics are quick-moving exercises which involve jumping or bouncing in order to make the working muscles alternate quickly between eccentric and concentric action. Examples of plyometric exercises include chest jumps, bench jumps, star jumps, squat jumps, burpees, hopping and bounding. They are only done if you are active in sports and your knee has virtually recovered full fitness. They can be used for 'fitness testing' for professional sports players, or as final-stage rehabilitation exercises leading to the return to playing.

Isokinetic muscle testing

Isokinetic machines provide an accommodating resistance which adapts to the weaker parts of a muscle's range. Technically called isokinetic dynamometers, they are used mainly for measuring concentric and eccentric muscle efficiency, although they can also be used for remedial and training exercise. Muscle measurements can be invaluable for identifying details of functional deficits in order to establish a precise remedial exercise programme, especially in the later stages of recovery from an injury.

Balance and co-ordination exercises

Balance exercises can be static or dynamic. They are best done barefoot, so that all the nerve mechanisms in the foot and upwards have to work without the support of a shoe. Standing still on one leg is the simplest version of static balance exercise. It can be made harder by closing your eyes, or by throwing and catching a ball. A progression is to stand on a mini-trampoline or wobble board, at first with eyes open, later with eyes closed. A slightly different kind of balance mechanism is trained by standing still on one leg while moving the other. Dynamic balance exercises can involve standing on one leg, bending and straightening the knee, going up and down on the toes, or combining these movements in sequence.

The simplest balance training exercises are usually introduced into the remedial programme as soon as you can stand on your injured leg. Special attention is paid to the recovery of good balance mechanisms following any serious derangement inside the knee, such as a cruciate ligament tear.

Stretching and mobilizing exercises

Stretching exercises are used to increase flexibility in muscles and tendons. There are many different theories about how to do it safely and effectively. I define safe stretching techniques very precisely. The muscle group is taken to its active limit, then given a slight over-pressure in the same direction. The muscles are relaxed so that the stretch is passive. There should be a very slight feeling of stretching. The stretched position can be held for a count of about six to ten, then the muscles are released to the starting position. Any strong sensation in the muscles, or any further movement, trying to stretch further from the already stretched position, is unlikely to improve the muscle length, and risks causing damage.

Mobilizing exercises help to increase a joint's freedom and range of movement. They involve gentle rhythmic bouncing movements, which help lubricate the joint. They can be done as free exercises, such as sitting

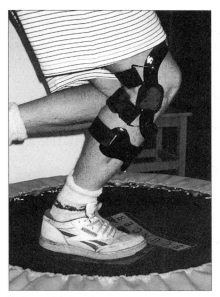

Doing weightbearing movements on the mini-trampoline trains the balance mechanisms

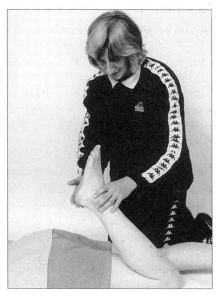

For safe stretching, the muscle group is taken to its active limit, and then slight over-pressure is applied

on a high bench and swinging your leg to bend and straighten the knee, or as assisted exercises with over-pressure, for instance lying on your stomach and rocking your foot towards your bottom to increase knee flexion, or sitting on the floor with your foot supported on a wedge and pressing rhythmically downwards on your thigh for better knee extension. An exercise bicycle can be used to improve knee flexion, if you sit and pedal without any resistance in an arc backwards and forwards to your limit each way. Once you can achieve a full turn backwards, you work to turn the pedals forwards. As the range of knee-bending improves, you gradually lower the saddle.

To prevent stiffness in the knee or its muscles, stretching and mobilizing exercises should be done daily, especially if you are sitting for most of the day. Passive stretching exercises should be done 'cold' in the morning or as the first part of a warm-up prior to exercise or sport, with care not to stretch beyond the muscles' limits, which are less than when the muscles are warmed up. The stretching should be repeated at the end of the warm-up, after any exercise session or warm-down routine, and last thing in the evening. The mobilizing exercises can be done at any time during the day, and alongside the passive stretching exercises.

Pool exercises

Exercise in water provides a variety of benefits, without causing any jarring in the knees. Hydrotherapy, or remedial exercises in water, may be part of your physiotherapy programme, although it is more readily available in European countries other than Britain. The water is used to create different exercise effects. Lying supported by floats, buoyancy assists upward movements and you can move your legs across the surface of the water, for instance adducting and abducting your hips, to gain mobility and co-ordination. You can use the water as resistance to downward movements, for instance by 'cycling': if you lie on your back the gluteal and hamstring muscles are resisted, the front-thigh muscles assisted, and vice versa on your front. The faster you move in the water, the greater the resistance provided by the turbulence.

Swimming is good for generalized fitness. In most knee problems breast-stroke swimming causes pain, but crawl and back-stroke are usually painless. Walking in the shallow end can help your balance and co-ordination, and is a good way of recovering confidence in weightbearing after a major injury or operation. A 'wet-vest' which provides buoyancy can allow you to simulate running in the water.

You may find it easier to move your knee in the water than on land, but take care not to do too much in any one session. Always do less than you think you can, so that you can build up the exercise programme gradually without setbacks. Exercise in water is very tiring, so you should not do too much at first, and you should rest lying down for at least ten minutes after the session.

ALTERNATIVE TRAINING

The remedial exercise programme is usually constructed to include an element of generalized fitness training for the heart and lungs (cardiorespiratory system) and for the uninjured parts of the body. The level of this training depends on the patient's current fitness and aspirations, so it is very limited for the older patient who is generally inactive, but very demanding for the young sports player who needs to prevent any major loss of fitness during the recovery period from a knee problem. The training programme may include various elements, such as speed, endurance and anaerobic training, as preparation for specific sports. Aerobic training is commonly used both for general fitness training and as a background to sports.

Aerobic training may be done using a circuit of exercises involving the uninjured parts of the body, or, once the knee has recovered sufficiently,

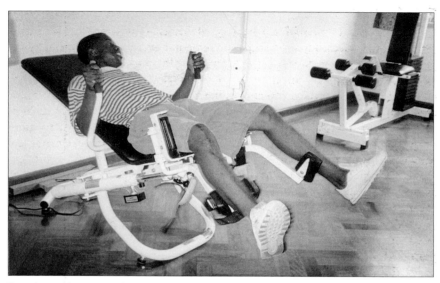

Exercise equipment can be used for alternative training. The Hydrafitness system provides concentric exercise for opposing muscle groups such as the hip abductors and adductors, and can be used for aerobic training

machines which work the legs, such as an exercise or road bicycle, stepper (Stair-climber or Stair-master), or rowing ergometer. The patient who smokes should try to break the habit, or at least not give in to the temptation to smoke more because of boredom, idleness or depression. It can be encouraging to be aware that a two-hour gap between a cigarette and energetic exercise can increase one's lung efficiency by about a third.

BASIC REMEDIAL AND PROTECTIVE EXERCISES FOR THE KNEE

Remedial and protective exercises should never cause or increase pain. Exercises are chosen and progressed according to the state of your knee at any given moment. The programme always includes exercises for all aspects of the knee, to create muscle balance, with specific emphasis on any areas of special weakness or inadequacy.

The exercises listed here cover most knee activities which are likely to be disrupted through injury or pain. Exercises 1–11 provide a basic programme for vastus medialis obliquus recovery, knee joint stability and mobility, and they can be used as a remedial and protective system for almost any knee injury or pain condition. These exercises can be used to start the rehabilitation process, and for long-term protection of the knees. Of the other exercises (12–25), some are done specifically for certain injuries, and some only at certain stages of the rehabilitation programme. After full recovery, all of the exercises can be used as a general protective programme for the legs.

1. Vastus medialis obliquus control, sitting down

Sit with your legs straight in front of you, on the floor or on the edge of a chair with your leg straight and your heel on the floor. Twitch your thigh muscles very slightly to move your kneecap upwards a little on the thigh, with as little activity as possible in the outer thigh muscles. Hold for a count of two, then release for a count of five. Repeat 5–10 times.

Note: This movement requires concentration, not effort. If you find it difficult, limit yourself to three repetitions only at a time, and repeat every hour or two. Once you can perform the movement accurately, repeat it frequently throughout the day. Try to incorporate it into your daily life, especially if you sit at a desk for much of the day. Once you are aware of how to release the kneecap, this exercise will help you to relax your thigh muscles and prevent involuntary tension.

2. Knee hyperextension, sitting down

Sitting with your legs straight in front of you, on the floor or on the edge of a chair with your heel on the floor, foot at right angles to your leg and

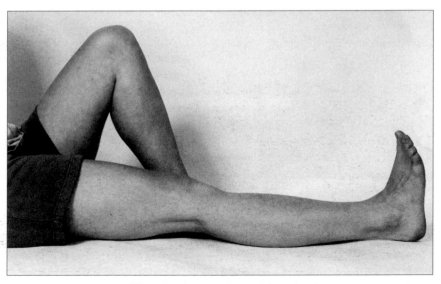

Locking the knee straight. (The other knee can be straight or bent)

toes relaxed, straighten your knee as hard as you can. Hold for a count of two, relax for a count of five. Repeat 5–10 times.

Note: Try to do this exercise frequently during the day. Sitting on the edge of an upright chair, leg straight with your heel on the floor, you can lock your knee while sitting at a desk.

3. Side-lying hip abduction

Lie on one side with your hips well forward, body straight and feet at right angles to your legs, toes relaxed; lift your upper leg up towards the ceiling, keeping the knee locked straight. Hold for a count of two, slowly lower, and relax for a count of five. Repeat 10–12 times.

Note: Make sure your hips are fully extended and your lower back slightly arched. Keep your head straight, and do not look down towards your feet. If your hips and trunk are bent, you will bring the leg forwards and use the muscles at the front of the hip instead of those at the side. If your legs are uncomfortable when they touch each other, use a small pillow between your knees for cushioning.

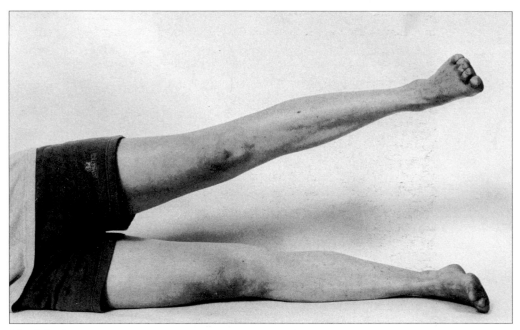

Hip abduction

4. Prone-lying hip extension

Lying on your front, with your toes pointing downwards in line with your leg, straighten your knee and lift your leg upwards behind you a little way. Lock your knee straight again, hold for a count of two, slowly lower to the floor and relax for a count of five. Repeat 10–20 times.

Note: You can only lift your leg about 15 degrees at the most, as this is the normal limit of hip extension. If you try to lift your leg any higher, you will curve your back. If your back aches when you do this exercise, place a pillow under your abdomen and make sure you are not lifting your leg too high. When the leg is behind you, it is all too easy to lose the feeling of extension at the knee, and carelessly let the knee bend slightly. This is why you must concentrate on locking the knee straight after you have lifted the leg up.

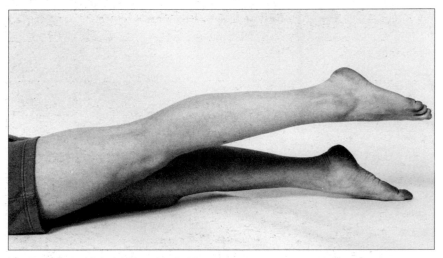

Hip extension with locked knee

5. Prone-lying active knee-bending

Lying on your front, bend your knee quite quickly as far as you can comfortably, then straighten it out slowly and relax. Repeat 20 times.

Note: If your kneecap aches because of the direct pressure on it, place a folded towel under your thigh to lift the knee off the floor. Make sure you straighten the knee fully and let all the muscles relax completely before repeating the movement. To improve hamstring strength you can use progressively increasing weights on your foot or around your ankle.

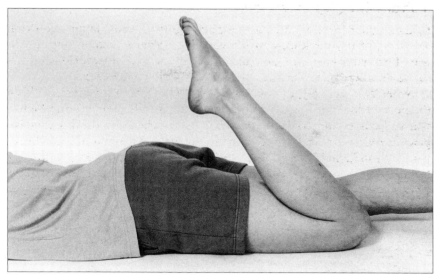

Active knee-bending

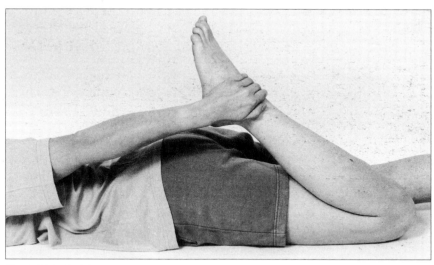

Front-thigh stretch

6. Prone-lying front-thigh stretch

Lying on your front, bend your knee as far as it can go actively. Hold your ankle with your hand and gently pull to bring your heel slightly further in towards your bottom. Hold for a count of six, then relax and let the leg straighten out again. Repeat 5–10 times.

Note: Put a folded towel under your thigh if your kneecap aches in the front-lying position. Do not over-stretch. The feeling of stretching should be very mild, and the movement should be no more than a few degrees. If you have difficulty reaching your foot with your hand, put a belt round your ankle so that you can pull gently on the ends of the belt.

7. Standing balance

Stand on one leg, preferably barefoot, and hold your balance for as long as possible. Repeat 3 times on each leg.

Note: Make sure your back is straight, and your pelvis level. Relax your toes and do not let them grip the ground. Stand close to a support in case you overbalance, but do not lean on it. If it is harder to balance on one side than the other, do extra repetitions for the more difficult side.

8. Standing hip abduction

Standing on one leg, preferably barefoot, lift the other leg sideways with control. Keeping the knee straight, lower the leg again without putting it to the floor, then repeat the sideways lift. Repeat 5–20 times on each side.

Note: Keep your back straight, head up, and make sure your pelvis is level throughout the movement. Relax your toes. You may need to steady yourself with your hand to keep your balance, but do not lean on a support. This exercise is especially important if there is any weakness or incoordination stemming from the hip. If you find it more difficult to do this movement correctly on one side than the other, do more repetitions on the difficult side, but take care to do every repetition with full control.

9. Calf raise

Stand on one leg and go up and down on your toes with control, keeping your knee straight and your toes as relaxed as possible. Repeat 5–20 times on each leg.

Note: Try to do this movement as slowly as you can while maintaining your balance. Control the reverse movement carefully. If it is more difficult on one leg than the other, do more repetitions for the more difficult side.

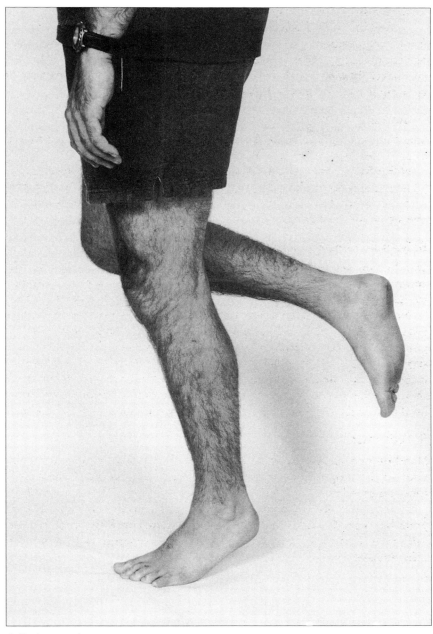

Calf raise exercise

10. Calf stretch

Stand with one leg behind the other, legs shoulder-width apart, feet in line facing forwards, front leg bent, back leg straight. Gently bend the front leg a little, until you feel a slight stretch on the back leg. Hold the stretch absolutely still for a count of six, then relax completely. Repeat 5–10 times.

Note: If one calf feels tight relative to the other, take care not to over-stretch it: take it only to the limit where you feel a mild sensation. Do more repetitions for the tighter side. Calf stretching should be done regularly, before and after any exercises or training, and morning and evening.

11. Hamstring stretch standing

Standing with one leg straight in front of you with the heel resting on a low support, lean forwards gently, keeping your head up, back straight. Hold for a count of six, then relax completely. Repeat 5–10 times.

Note: Do not over-stretch by pulling your head downwards or forcing your hands towards your toes. You should only feel a very mild sensation of stretch. If one leg is tighter than the other, do extra repetitions for the shorter hamstrings. Stretch regularly, as for calf stretching.

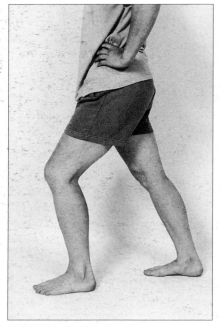

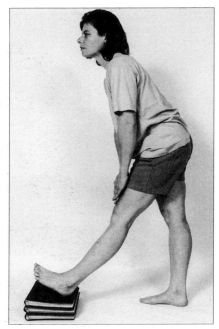

Calf stretch for right leg

Hamstring stretch, standing

12. Thigh adductor stretch standing

Standing with your legs apart, shift your weight slightly towards one side, and lean sideways over the other side to feel the stretch down the inner thigh. Hold for a count of six, then relax completely. Repeat 5–10 times.

Note: Do not over-stretch, and take care not to bend or twist your trunk as you lean sideways. Stretch regularly, as for calf stretching.

13. Isometric hamstring exercise

Sitting on a chair with your heel against the chair-leg, knee bent to at least a right angle, foot pointing forwards, press your heel back against the chair-leg to tense your hamstring muscles. Hold for a count of two, then relax completely for a count of five. Repeat 5 times.

Note: This exercise is used to correct weakness in the hamstrings, especially after surgery for cruciate ligament tears. For a hyperextending knee, the exercise can be repeated every hour, using increasing degrees of flexion.

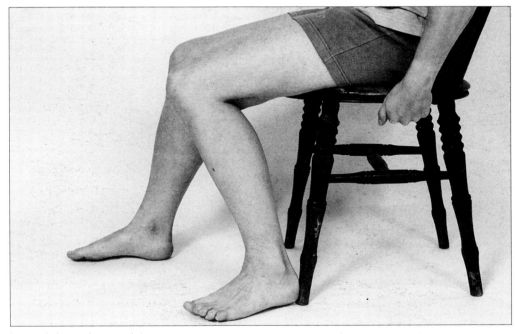

Isometric hamstring exercise

14. Isometric biceps femoris exercise

Sitting on a chair with your knee bent to a right angle or more, heel against the chair-leg and foot turned outwards, press your heel against the chair-leg to increase tension in the outer hamstring muscle. Hold for a count of two, relax completely for a count of five. Repeat 5 times.

Note: This exercise is used to correct imbalance between the inner two hamstrings and biceps femoris, especially in cases of anterior cruciate ligament injury.

15. Vastus medialis obliquus control, standing up

Standing with your legs straight, twitch your thigh muscles very slightly to move your kneecap upwards a little on the thigh, with as little activity as possible in the outer thigh muscles. Hold for a count of two, then release for a count of five. Repeat 3–5 times.

Note: You may need to stand in front of a mirror to check the movement and release of the kneecap at first. Once you have full control over the vastus medialis obliquus, you can practise this exercise whenever you are standing up during the day. It is a good way of checking whether your muscles are tensing up unconsciously during your normal activities.

16. Heel-supported knee extension

Sitting with your legs straight in front of you, place a small block or rolled towel under your heel, straighten your knee downwards firmly,

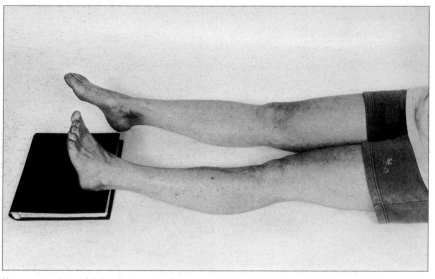

Knee extension with heel supported

with control, keeping your foot pointing vertically upwards, toes relaxed. Hold for a count of two, relax for a count of five. Repeat 5–10 times.

Note: If this exercise causes pain over the front of the knee, rub ice on it. If this relieves the pain, the exercise can be repeated. This movement is generally not used if the knee hyperextends excessively.

17. Knee hyperextension with hip adduction, sitting down

Sitting with your legs straight in front of you on the floor or on the edge of a chair with your heel on the floor, place a block or medicine ball between your feet, then press your knees as straight as you can, while pressing your feet gently inwards against the block or medicine ball. Hold for a count of two, release for a count of five. Repeat 5–10 times.

Note: Do not exert forceful or excessive pressure for any element of this exercise. Keep your feet pointing upwards, symmetrically.

18. Prone-lying knee extension

Lying on your stomach with your foot at right angles to your leg, balancing on the balls of your feet, straighten your knee as fully as possible in a controlled way; hold for a count of two, then relax completely for a count of five. Repeat 5–10 times.

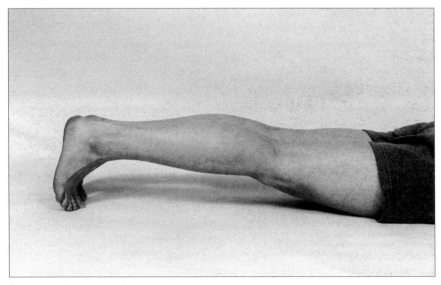

Prone-lying knee extension

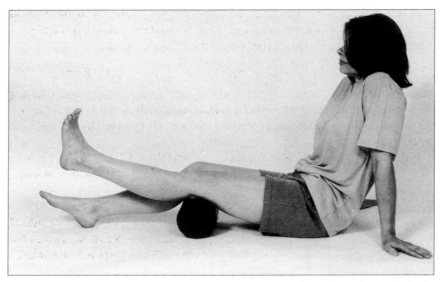

Knee extension over a wedge

19. Knee extension over a wedge

Sitting with your legs straight in front of you, and a small wedge or rolled towel under your knee, straighten your knee firmly for a count of two, slowly lower, and relax for a count of five. Repeat 5-10 times.

Note: It is vital to straighten the knee fully. Once you can perform the exercise correctly with ease, you can progress by using ankle weights or a weights boot with gradually increasing load. You can also increase the repetitions to three sets of 10–15 in stages.

20. Vastus medialis obliquus fine-tune control, sitting down

Sitting with your legs straight, twitch your kneecap upwards without activating your outer thigh muscles, relax, then twitch the kneecap again. See if you can perform six repetitions of twitch-release rhythmically in quick succession.

Note: You will only be able to perform this movement properly when you have very good control of the VMO and its controlling nerve.

21. Straight-leg-raise

Sitting on the floor with your legs straight in front of you, turn one leg outwards, lock the knee straight and lift the leg upwards a little way, keeping the knee locked; hold for a count of two, slowly lower and relax completely. Repeat 10–20 times.

Note: This exercise can only be done properly when you have good control of the VMO. When you can do it accurately, you can progress by using gradually increasing weights over your foot or ankle.

22. Vastus medialis obliquus fine-tune control, standing up

Standing with your legs straight, twitch your kneecap upwards without activating your outer thigh muscles, relax, then twitch the kneecap again. See if you can perform six repetitions of twitch-release rhythmically in quick succession.

Note: This exercise requires excellent control of the VMO. It is a very useful way of making sure the VMO is not tense during normal standing.

23. Hip abductor stretch sitting

Sitting on the floor, bend one knee and place the foot beside the outer side of the other knee; with the opposite hand, press the bent knee gently across the other leg, hold for a count of six, then relax completely. Repeat 5–10 times.

24. Dynamic balance

Standing on one leg, go up on your toes and straighten your knee, put your heel down and bend your knee, then repeat the sequence 5–10 times without putting the other leg down.

Note: Stand close to a support, in case you overbalance. Keep your back as straight as possible. Do only as many repetitions as you can with full control.

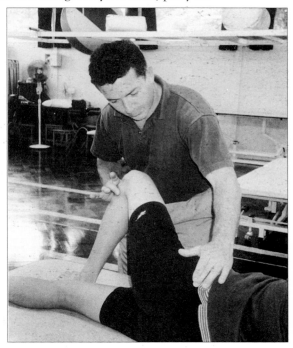

Leg position for hip abductor stretching. The stretch can be done lying down or sitting up.

25. Squat

Standing on your toes with your feet slightly apart, back straight and head up, bend your knees as far as you comfortably can, straighten up and lock the knees, then relax and go back on to your heels. Repeat 5–10 times.

Note: Support yourself with your hands at first, for confidence. It is easier to do this movement quickly than slowly. As your strength and confidence improve, you should go down more slowly, with full control. Stay on your toes as you go down.

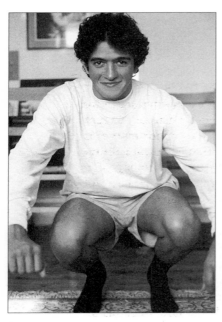

Squatting is an important goal. Imbalance may be corrected by watching the movement in a mirror

Safety tips during rehabilitation

- Do your prescribed remedial exercises accurately and frequently
- Do not try to work through pain
- If in doubt, always refer to your practitioner
- Progress your activities according to your practitioner's guidelines
- Do not attempt activities which stress or test your knee until you and your practitioner are confident you are fit enough

Coping with knee problems

11

First aid

Training in basic first-aid techniques is a must for everyone. It is rare for a doctor or qualified paramedic to be on hand when an accident happens. Knowing what to do when faced with major or minor injuries is especially important for people who have a particular responsibility towards others. Parents and teachers should be capable of coping with children's accidents. Physical education teachers, sports coaches and referees are all likely to be faced with injuries among sports players at some time. In the workplace, there should always be someone on duty who is capable of administering first aid if necessary.

The first priority in first aid is to deal with any life-threatening factors with appropriate resuscitation techniques. Certain types of trauma to the knee must be treated as emergencies, including fractures in the thigh-bone or shin-bone, dislocation of the main (tibiofemoral) knee joint and wounds involving the joint. The first-aider should know how to recognize these injuries and minimize the dangers of infections or further displacement of broken bones. Bleeding in association with a knee injury must be stopped by continuous compression with sterile dressings or clean material. Major arteries pass through the knee area, so if large amounts of blood are being pumped out through a wound, there is a strong risk that the victim will go into clinical shock.

The majority of traumatic knee injuries are not dangerous, although they are usually very painful. Even if immediate hospital treatment is not needed, the patient should be advised to seek treatment, preferably through a general practitioner in the first instance. The first-aid priority is to reduce pain and swelling as quickly as possible, and the simplest and safest solution is ICE – ice applications, compression and elevation.

ICE APPLICATIONS

The purpose of applying ice is to stimulate a healthy flow of blood through the injured area, and to prevent any increase of internal bruising or bleeding, which might result after the initial impact of the injury.

Ice can be applied in different ways. A simple method is to massage round the injured area with an ice cube. Ice cups can be prepared for 'cryomassage' by placing crushed ice or water in a paper beaker and putting it into the freezer. When it is needed, the top edge of the beaker can be cut away to leave a rim of ice ready to apply. You can put crushed ice into a plastic bag to make an ice pack, or use a ready-made chemical ice pack, but you must protect the skin with a damp towel or at least some olive or baby oil. As an alternative to ice, you can use a flannel soaked in cold water as a cold wrap round the knee, but you will have to keep rinsing it under the cold tap to prevent it from heating up and losing its effect.

There are different theories about how long the ice or cold compress should be applied. I prefer to use the ice for a short period, anything from about two to ten minutes, and to repeat the application at regular intervals, according to need. Some people advocate immersing the knee in ice for up to an hour or more. In all cases, you must watch the skin for signs of damage. Following ice application, it is normal for the skin to turn pink in a Caucasian, or darker in a dark-skinned person. If the skin becomes irritated, brittle and sore from the ice, do not try to apply any more until it has recovered.

COMPRESSION AND SUPPORT

Compression can be achieved with a tubular bandage or sleeve, or layers of cotton wool wrapped round the joint interspersed with crêpe bandaging. To restrict joint movement even further, taping, a splint or a plaster cast may be used. The knee is usually fixed in the straight position, although in certain cases it may be kept bent.

Total immobility for the joint is only advisable if absolutely necessary, and for the minimum period possible, because of the detrimental effect it has on the circulation and the muscles surrounding the joint. An enclosing sleeve type of bandage, similarly, should only be used when necessary, and it should be removed whenever possible, for instance when you are sitting with the leg supported. If it is left on for too long it may inhibit the knee muscles, especially vastus medialis obliquus.

If a bandage or splint is applied to your knee, it must extend from at least halfway up your calf to halfway up your thigh, or even from your ankle to near the top of your thigh. If it only covers the knee joint itself, it will probably ruck up to become too tight and create unwanted pressure. When your knee is bandaged, you must check the circulation in your leg at regular intervals. Squeeze your big toe to see whether the colour returns to it quickly when you let go. If you notice that your foot is an abnormal colour, or that you are experiencing cramp in your leg muscles, you should loosen or remove the bandage or splint, and refer to your practitioner if the cramp does not recover immediately.

ELEVATION

In order to help the circulatory flow, the leg should be supported with the foot raised above the level of the hip. The whole leg should rest on a pillow or cushioned support. If only the heel is supported, there will be painful pressure at the back of the knee. Changing position helps, especially during the early stages of recovery from an injury or operation. If you can lie on your sound side comfortably, you should place a pillow between your knees. If you lie on the affected side, keep the knee clear of pressure from the other leg: you can stretch the affected leg behind or in front of you, and support the sound leg on a pillow. If you are able to turn on to your stomach, you can put pillows under your abdomen and lower legs for comfort, to lie in this position for at least short periods.

EMERGENCY HOSPITAL TREATMENT

In an emergency, if you have been taken to the casualty department following a severe knee injury, you may be assessed and treated by the casualty officer, an accident surgeon or an orthopaedic surgeon. The decision may be taken to operate on your knee immediately, subject to your consent, or you may be admitted to hospital for observation and bed-rest. Try to give the surgeon an accurate picture of exactly what happened to your knee in the accident, where it hurts, whether you have pain anywhere else apart from the knee, and whether you can move your leg at all with or without pain. The surgeon also needs to know when you last ate or drank anything, and whether you are allergic to any particular drugs.

If you are to be allowed home, your knee will probably be bandaged or put into a plaster cast, and you will be given crutches to use, or at least a walking stick. Your progress will then be monitored by the orthopaedic specialist, in case you need surgery at a later stage.

IF YOU NEED AN OPERATION AT A LATER STAGE

Except in an emergency, there may be a delay from a few days to several months from the time you are advised to have an operation to the time it happens. You should use the time to prepare yourself physically and mentally for the operation. Don't just wait in the hope that the operation will solve everything on its own. The better prepared you are, the easier and more complete your recovery is likely to be.

Remedial exercises and fitness work

As part of your physical preparation you should be doing remedial exercises every day. The surgeon may have a special regime which you will be shown by the physiotherapist in the surgeon's team. You may be able to do your exercises under the supervision of the physiotherapist individually or with other patients in a 'knee class' in the clinic or hospital. This can be a great help to your motivation, but you must also do your exercises at home.

The fitter your heart and lungs, the better you will cope with the anaesthetic. You must look after your circulation carefully before the operation, and establish good habits of circulatory care to avoid the risk of blood clots forming after the operation. Try to do some aerobic training, such as swimming, cycling, rowing or circuit training, depending on what you can do without irritating your knee.

Breathing exercises

Controlled breathing exercises should be part of your daily routine, especially if you are a smoker. If you smoke, you should stop, or at least cut down. The less you smoke in the hours, days and weeks before your operation, the more you reduce your risk of getting a chest infection after the anaesthetic. The simplest form of breathing exercise is to take a deep breath in, concentrating on feeling your ribs swell outwards, then breathe out for slightly longer than normal, without blowing hard, so that you feel your ribs sinking inwards. Repeat this exercise about three to five times once or twice a day, but do not try to do too many repetitions at a time, because you may get dizzy. You need to be comfortable, so that you can perform the breathing exercises without tensing your neck and shoulders. You can sit with your elbows resting on your knees or a table, or you can lie down.

Diet

Your diet should consist of regular, healthy, varied and well-balanced meals. Do not go on a 'crash diet', even if you are worried that your weight might increase because you cannot do your normal levels of exercise. Control your weight by avoiding snacks and 'comfort foods' like crisps and chocolates, and maintaining an exercise programme. Avoid drinking excessive tea, coffee, juices or alcohol, or preferably cut them out completely. If you have particular problems relating to diet, you must consult a dietician or nutritionist, preferably through your general practitioner.

Mental preparation

Mental preparation is vital. You need to be calm and relaxed as you go in for the operation, and you need to be thinking positively about your recovery. If you have any worries about the operation itself, discuss them with your surgeon or general practitioner. If it is difficult to get to see the surgeon, write a letter expressing your concerns and asking for reassurance.

If you are stressed for other reasons, try to get appropriate counselling, and you can ask your general practitioner for guidance about this. Relaxation classes may help. You must make sure that you have yourself and your environment under control. Rationalize your activities so that you avoid unnecessary commitments or a frantic last-minute rush to get things done before you go into hospital. You must be free of worries, such as responsibilities to family, business concerns, exams or personal problems.

Preparing for an operation

- Do your remedial exercises conscientiously every day
- If you smoke, stop, or at least cut down
- Practise breathing exercises regularly
- Keep yourself fit with exercises and/or aerobic training
- Maintain as varied and healthy a diet as possible
- Drink plenty of water all day, every day
- During your daily activities, keep your body moving as much as possible
- Wear sensible shoes and clothes, to avoid circulatory constriction
- Plan your time and activities before and after the operation carefully
- Avoid fatigue, stress or pressurizing yourself
- Rest and relax for a period every day

Getting ready on the day of the operation

- Check that you have packed the clothes and toiletries you need
- Take some reading material or pastimes in case you have to wait
- Do not smoke at all on the day of the operation
- Do not eat or drink anything after the time specified when your fast should start
- Make sure you have completed all necessary tasks before you go into hospital
- Be calm, rest and think positively
- Practise controlled breathing exercises
- Do your remedial exercises

Recovering from the anaesthetic

After an operation, all the surgical wounds have to heal, you have to get over the anaesthetic, and your knee has to recuperate. The main complications which can set in post-operatively are wound infections, blood clot formation and chest infections.

Even if the operation is over very quickly and the anaesthetic has been short-lasting, you should allow several days to recover. Your knee may feel painless and mobile, but you may still feel surprisingly tired, mainly because of the anaesthetic. Some people suffer more ill-effects from the anaesthetic than others. Hard physical effort for sport or manual work is out of the question until your surgeon gives you the all-clear. Don't try to rush back to normal activities, especially if they involve skills like driving or concentrated precision work. Wait until you feel ready. Even after the most minor operation this is likely to take at least a week.

The anaesthetic can have a bad effect on your chest, so you should do controlled breathing exercises for as long as you are not fully mobile. Try to cough up any phlegm that you feel rattling in your chest. If your chest feels tight or if you notice that the phlegm is green, you should refer to your doctor in case you have an infection which needs treatment.

Care for the circulation, wounds and swelling

The risk of blood clots forming in your knee or leg will be present for some time after the operation, the more so if you are unable to walk and move around freely. An untreated blood clot can be extremely dangerous, even life-threatening, although mercifully this is rare. If you notice a deep burning sensation anywhere in your leg you should refer to your doctor or surgeon urgently.

Depending on the type of operation, your knee may show only the tiny entry holes (technically known as portals) of the arthroscope, or a scar where the surgeon has cut through the skin to reach the joint. The wound may be sealed with stitches which are self-dissolving or by stitches that need to be removed. In the first ten to fourteen days after the operation while the wound is healing, you should take care not to let it get dirty. It should be covered with a clean dressing at all times.

Ask your surgeon or doctor at what stage you can start showering, taking a bath or using a communal pool. You may be able to take a shower if you protect your knee from the water with a plastic covering, but you may not be allowed to take a bath. Once the wound is fully healed, you can safely get into the bath. If the scar is still a little sore, or not quite healed, it can help to put salt into the bath-water. You must wait until the wound has closed completely before using communal swimming pools or jacuzzis, as even the tiniest open wound can get infected. If you notice any signs of skin irritation, soreness or odour in the operation wound, you must refer to your surgeon or doctor immediately.

Most knee operations leave the knee swollen afterwards. Especially in the first few days, the swelling should be controlled with ice packs or cold compresses and supportive bandaging. The bandaging may be removed at night. It is discarded as soon as possible so that it is not worn out of habit: to do this inhibits the knee muscles.

Post-operative rehabilitation

The best results from an operation will be achieved if you allow enough time to complete a full rehabilitation programme. The operation is only the first step towards recovery. It cannot restore functional activities to your knee: only specific exercises can do that.

Most orthopaedic surgeons recommend physiotherapy for their patients before and after surgery. The physiotherapist may be part of the clinical team in a hospital, or may be independent of the surgeon. In some cases, the physiotherapist may observe the operation, but, if not, details of what has been done are provided by the surgeon together with any special instructions relating to the rehabilitation.

The details of the treatment are usually left to the physiotherapist, who informs the surgeon immediately and refers the patient back if there are any problems. The surgeon usually monitors the patient at intervals, and may even continue to review the patient once a year indefinitely if the problem was especially complicated and likely to have longer-term consequences.

CIRCULATORY CARE

Looking after your circulation should be a routine part of your normal daily life, as it is important for your general health. Any slight restriction of the blood flow in your legs can lead to problems even in the absence of injury. Constriction can make your feet and legs swell up, or cause extra congestion in varicose veins. A small degree of dehydration can cause muscle cramp and make the muscles more prone to strains and tears. Smoking cigarettes, cigars or a pipe is detrimental to the circulation. Circulatory care measures are especially important if you have to travel by air, particularly on long flights, because of the pressure on your legs due to altitude.

After any injury or operation, the fluid flow in the knee is disrupted, so circulatory care measures should start immediately. You need a good flow of fresh blood through the leg to help healing and to prevent congestion. The veins through which de-oxygenated blood is pushed back towards the heart depend on the pumping action of your leg muscles to keep the flow going, so if your normal leg movements are restricted, you have to find other ways of keeping the blood circulating.

For detailed advice about how to look after your circulation, you should ask your doctor or practitioner for guidance. The basic principles are to avoid harmful constriction and to stimulate a healthy throughput of blood.

A vital element of circulatory care is an adequate intake of plain water. The adult needs about ten glasses of water daily, and the child may need even more, as children dehydrate more easily than adults. Other types of drink, such as tea, coffee, fizzy drinks, juices and alcohol are not really helpful for fluid replacement, and in some cases they contribute to dehydration. Water should be taken from the morning onwards, on its own and as an accompaniment to food or other types of drink. Good water-drinking habits must start in childhood, as adults who have never drunk much water find it increasingly difficult to drink any as they get older, and this can have a disastrous effect on the kidneys.

Anything which blocks the blood flow in either direction will cause harm, so you must avoid constriction in any part of the leg. Do not wear tight trousers, socks, garters, stockings, tights or shoes, and avoid wearing tight clothing or belts round your waist. If your leg has been put into a plaster cast, refer back to your practitioner immediately if you notice that it is creating pressure or tightness against your leg, as the plaster should be removed urgently. Never rest either leg on a hard surface, or cross your legs at the knees or ankles.

If you are on bed-rest following an injury or operation, you should avoid direct pressure on any part of your body. Keep moving your legs, arms and trunk as much as you can. The physiotherapist usually sets out a programme of isometric exercises to maintain muscle tone, to be done hourly.

In any situation, avoid sitting or standing still for any length of time with the leg down, as gravity makes fluid pool into the lower leg, creating congestion. Support the injured leg up, resting on a soft cushion or pillow. Whether lying down, sitting or standing, keep your foot moving whenever possible. If you can move your knee without creating pain, you should bend and straighten it gently. Even in a plaster cast, you may be able to tighten and relax the quadriceps muscles, and to move your leg from the hip without problems or pain.

If you can put any pressure through the sole of your foot, you can rub the soft central part over a golf ball or foot massager. This is a powerful stimulus to the blood flow, and it helps reduce swelling and prevent fluid from gathering in the leg below the knee. If you cannot bend your knee to put the foot to the floor, you can perhaps fix a wooden foot massager so that you can stretch your leg to it horizontally, for instance at the foot of your bed. This type of foot self-massage can be done every half-hour or so.

If you have a localized painful or bruised area over the knee, especially following direct trauma such as a knock, it can be helpful to massage round it gently with a heparinoid cream, or apply a compress soaked in arnica lotion to it, held in place by a light bandage.

Generalized movements help your overall circulatory flow, so lift your arms up and down, or swing them around in big circles as often as possible, standing up or sitting down. Exercise your uninjured leg as much as you can to keep the muscles, nerve systems and circulation going. If you are able to get into the bath, gentle leg movements in warm water are a great help for the circulation, but do not have the water too hot.

Varicose veins will become more prominent and possibly more painful if the circulatory flow is compromised. Varicose veins are usually inherited, but they can also appear as the result of a leg injury, often reflecting circulatory constriction through carelessness. It is as well to observe the general principles of circulatory care indefinitely as a precaution against later problems, especially if you already have circulatory problems such as varicose veins.

CRUTCHES

In the early stages of recovery after a bad injury or operation, you may have to use crutches to keep the pressure off your painful knee. The crutches should be used until you can walk comfortably without a limp.

The crutches should be the right height, so that you do not have to

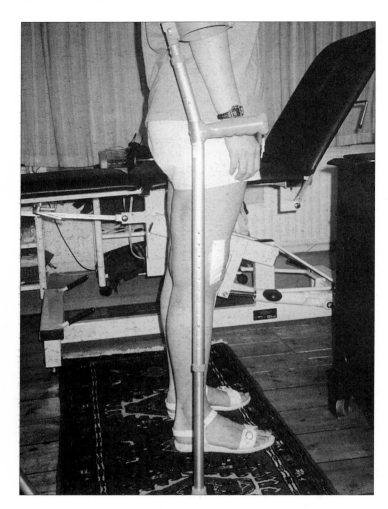

Measuring the crutches: the crutch handle should be level with the wrist

stoop as you push down on the handles. If you use axillary crutches, which come up to just below the armpits, you must not rest your armpits on top of them, as you can damage major nerves, leading to numbness, tingling and eventually partial paralysis in your hands. If this happens, the nerves usually recover given time, but it is a slow process. The correct way to use axillary crutches is to keep your head up, back straight, and press the tops of the crutches inwards against the sides of your chest as you take your weight through your hands. Elbow crutches which reach up to the mid-part of your upper arm are easier to use than axillary crutches, so in Britain the majority of patients use these. When you walk

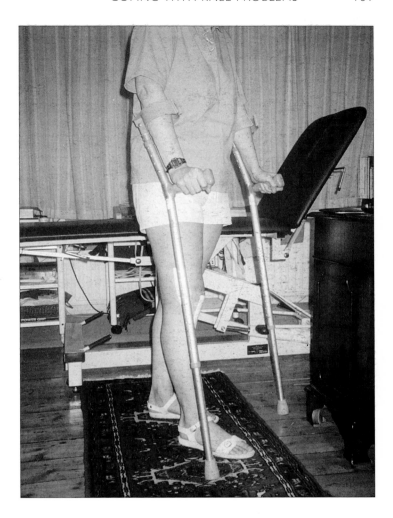

Walking with crutches
partially weightbearing, the
injured leg and crutches
move together

with crutches, take care not to place the crutches too far in front of you, especially if the ground is wet or slippery.

If you cannot take weight through your painful leg, press down on the crutch handles and swing your legs through between the crutches, landing on your sound leg between the crutches or a little way in front of them. Going up stairs, balance your weight between the crutches, place your sound leg on the step above, bring the crutches up beside you and repeat the process. Never try to put the crutches up on a step in front of you. Going down, the process is reversed, so you put the crutches down on to the next step first and then bring the sound leg on to the same step. If there is a banister, you may be able to use one crutch and the more stable support of the rail. As stairs can be quite difficult to negotiate using crutches, you may find it easier at home to go up and down stairs sitting on your bottom and manoeuvring your bodyweight using your sound leg and your arms.

If you can take some weight through the painful leg, there are two ways of using crutches for normal walking. At first it may be easier to put the crutches in front of you, place the painful leg alongside the crutches, press down on to your hands and take the sound leg through in front of you. Once you are used to the crutches, you can move crutches and painful leg simultaneously.

As your knee recovers, you may graduate to using one crutch or a stick, which should be held in the opposite hand to the painful knee. If you put the stick or crutch on the same side, you will lean on it and risk causing constriction in your hip or lower back on that side. Use the stick as you take weight through your painful leg, so that your bodyweight is evenly balanced.

GETTING ABOUT WITH A KNEE PROBLEM

Your mobility is inevitably impaired when you have a bad knee, and you must plan any kind of journey with care. Avoid walking too far, on rough ground, or up and down lots of stairs, until you know you can without pain or swelling. Take care when crossing busy roads: always use pedestrian crossings, and avoid the risk of having to rush. You must correct any tendency to limp. If you are walking flat-footed, concentrate on lifting your heel early and pushing off with your toes while walking, exaggerating the normal pattern. To improve walking up stairs, practise stepping up and down on to a low step at first, then on to a normal height.

Work out realistic and safe plans for travelling. Trying to go to work on the Underground in London's rush-hour, for instance, is definitely not advisable, even if your knee problem is minor. Sitting or standing, you will be cramped and in danger of being jostled. Any kind of public transport may be difficult to cope with. It can be hard to get on or off a bus or train, and sudden lurching movements may throw you off-balance and hurt your weakened knee. Allow plenty of time to get where you need to go. Make sure your hands are free. Carry the minimum possible and use a shoulder bag or rucksack.

In Britain your motor insurance is invalidated if you try to drive a car while you have any kind of disability which impairs your driving

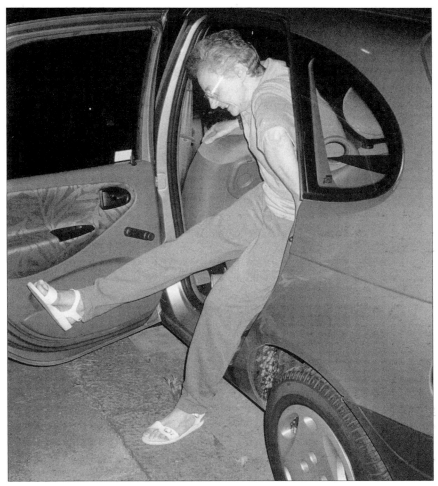

Getting into a car by sliding backwards on to the seat, keeping the injured leg straight

efficiency, unless you notify the authorities and pass a special driving test. One essential criterion for driving safety is your ability to do an emergency stop, so you should not even consider trying to drive if you have a painful right knee. On the other hand, if your left knee is disabled and you have an automatic car, you may be safe to drive as soon as you have practised on quiet safe roads and you feel confident. If in doubt, ask your doctor whether you are fit to drive or not.

When you are a passenger in a car, try to sit on the back seat and stretch your painful leg out on the seat, if possible. You may have to sit at an angle in order to use the seat belt properly. You should get into the car by sliding yourself on to the seat backwards from the door. This is much easier than trying to get in sideways in the usual way, unless the car has unusually spacious leg-room.

Narrow seats and lack of leg-room on aeroplanes can be a problem. If you have to go on a long flight, make sure that you have a fully reclining seat. Your doctor or specialist may be able to secure special arrangements for you on the basis of your disability, even though it is temporary.

Getting about with a knee problem is bound to be tiring, so allow time for rest periods lying down during the day to avoid excessive fatigue.

TIMESCALES FOR RECOVERY

Recovery from injuries

Basic healing time for damaged soft tissues which are capable of mending themselves is usually about ten days. However, if the tissue is constantly irritated, or if the damage is severe, the recovery time can be much longer. A badly strained or torn medial ligament, for instance, can take from three to six months, or even longer, to become painless.

Time has to be allowed for the remedial exercises to have their effect. It takes at least a month to derive any benefit from them, and proper adaptation to the remedial muscle work is only gained after about three months, even though good functional recovery may have been regained before that time. This is why it is worth practising the remedial exercises over an extended period.

Recovery from arthroscopy

Arthroscopy has significantly reduced the timescale for recovery from procedures such as cartilage removal (meniscectomy). Before arthroscopy became routine, the cartilage removal operation was much more invasive, and the scar itself required a recovery period of some weeks. After arthroscopy, unless any complications have arisen, you are normally walking about without crutches or a stick within a day. You may even be released from hospital on the same day as the operation. Most patients return to school, work and normal everyday activities within a few days. Professional soccer players are back on the field in a couple of weeks in many cases.

This apparently speedy recovery is deceptive and has its disadvantages. Your knee may feel virtually 'normal' within a couple of weeks of the operation, and you may be tempted to go straight back into full sporting activities. However, 'feeling normal' is not enough to guarantee that your knee is functioning fully. In fact it is impossible to regain total efficiency in the knee's co-ordinating mechanisms in such a short time.

I prefer patients to allow four to six weeks for rehabilitation before returning to sports which involve running, jumping, twisting, turning or contact. I apply this principle equally to professional and recreational sports players. It may seem a long time, but all too often the price paid for too early a return to punishing sports is more time off for secondary injuries, and, more seriously, long-term joint damage causing early painful arthritis. Too many professional competitors from sports like soccer, American football, basketball and ice hockey discover this to their cost long after their playing careers have ended.

Recovery after major surgery

After more invasive operations, such as cruciate ligament repair or total knee replacement, recovery is much slower. In most cases, the surgeon and rehabilitation team have a standard programme of remedial exercises and self-care which you should follow to the letter. You usually have to use crutches for the first period after the operation, until you can take your weight through the leg without discomfort. Bandaging or a special knee brace has to be used until the knee is comfortable and stable again. The time to full recovery varies according to the individual and ranges from three months up to nine months or longer.

Using knee supports

Following certain severe injuries such as cruciate ligament tears, you may need to use a protective support long-term for risky sports like skiing. The support should not be restrictive, but should be designed to protect the knee against abnormal stresses. The best protection is usually gained from an individually fitted brace, although these are inevitably expensive.

Supports which restrict knee movement should not be used in order to do activities that would otherwise be painful. Tubular bandages which encircle the knee should not be used for long periods or on a long-term basis.

Returning to normal activities

Be prepared to wait until you have achieved full functional recovery before testing your injured knee under pressure, however long it takes. If you try to stress the knee before it has recovered its protective mechanisms, compensation will make you vulnerable to re-injury or secondary injury somewhere else. You should recover stability, full movement and co-ordination in the injured knee, both when your weight is on the leg and when it is non-weightbearing.

Even if you are not active in your daily life, you should go through the stages of rehabilitation to make your knee fit. Remember that the knee is under stress even when you are not moving, and it can become painful through inactivity and neglect just as much as through excessive activity or accidents.

Returning to running

If running is part of your normal sports activities, it is important for your knee to be fit before you try to run again: you should be able to squat, or at least half-squat comfortably. Running jars the knees repetitively and tends to cause tightness in the muscles around the knee. Some protective

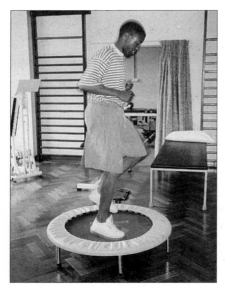

Running on the mini-trampoline provides co-ordination and aerobic training without jarring.

remedial knee exercises should be done before and after running sessions. Start on a treadmill, grass or soft flat ground, to minimize jarring, before going on to road or track. It is normal for the injured knee to swell slightly when you start running again. So long as the swelling reduces quickly with ice applications, you can continue running, but short distances only.

Never go running on consecutive days: a cautious and safe programme allows you to start by running once a week for the first month, twice a week for the second month, three times for the next month, building up gradually to four or five times a week running the distances of your choice. To prevent overuse injury syndromes and train dynamic co-ordination mechanisms in the knees, practise shuttle running, running sideways and backwards, running and turning, running with quick changes of direction, or running backwards in figure-of-eight patterns.

Musts for making your knee(s) better

- Accurate assessment and diagnosis
- Appropriate treatment
- Positive thinking
- Precise rehabilitation care

Bibliography

Much has been written about knees, clinically and scientifically. The following list of useful references is by no means exhaustive. It will be of interest to the reader who wishes to explore the subject in more technical detail.

Knee structure and function

Andriacchi, T P, Anderson, G B, Ortengren, R, Mikosz, R P, 1984, 'A study of factors influencing muscle activity about the knee joint', *Journal of Orthopaedic Research* 1: 266–275

Arnoczky, S P, Warren, R F, 1982, 'Microvasculature of the human meniscus', *American Journal of Sports Medicine* 10: 90–95

Aspden, R M, Yarker, Y E, Hukins, D W L, 1985, 'Collagen orientations in the meniscus of the knee joint', *Journal of Anatomy* 140: 371

Barrack, R L, Skinner, H B, Cook, S D, 1984, 'Proprioception of the knee joint: paradoxical effect of training', *American Journal of Physical Medicine* 63(4): 175–181

Biedert, R M, Stauffer, E, Friederich, N F, 1992, 'Occurrence of free nerve endings in the soft tissue of the knee joint: a histologic investigation', *American Journal of Sports Medicine* 20(4): 430–433

Bose, K, Kanagasuntheram, R, Osman, M B H, 1980, 'Vastus medialis oblique: an anatomic and physiologic study', *Orthopedics* 3: 880

Clark, C R, Ogden, J A, 1983, 'Development of the menisci of the human knee joint', *Journal of Bone and Joint Surgery* 65A: 530

Day, B, Mackenzie, W G, Shimm, S S, et al., 1985, 'The vascular and nerve supply of the human meniscus', *Arthroscopy* 1: 58

Francis, R S, Scott, D E, 1974, 'Hypertrophy of the vastus medialis in knee extension', *Physical Therapy* 54(10): 1066–1070

Ghosh, P, Taylor, T, Phil, D, 1987, 'The knee joint meniscus: A fibrocartilage of some distinction', *Clinical Orthopaedics and Related Research* 224: 52–63

Gollehan, D L, Torzilli, P A, Warren, R F, 1987, 'The role of the posterolateral and cruciate ligaments in the stability of the human knee', *Journal of Bone and Joint Surgery* 69B: 233

Grigg, P, 1994, 'Peripheral neural mechanisms in proprioception', *Journal of Sport Rehabilitation* 3(1): 2–17

Grood, E S, Stowers, S F, Noyes, F R, 1988, 'Limits of movement in the human knee', *Journal of Bone and Joint Surgery* 70B: 88

Jennings, A G, 1994, 'A proprioceptive role for the anterior cruciate ligament: a review of the literature', *Journal of Orthopaedic Rheumatology* 7: 3–13

Johansson, H, Sjolander, P, Sojka, P, 1991, 'A sensory role for the cruciate ligaments', *Clinical Orthopaedics and Related Research* 268: 161–177

Kennedy, J C, Alexander, I J, Hayes, K C, 1982, 'Nerve supply of the human knee and its functional importance', *American Journal of Sports Medicine* 10: 329–335

Lieb, F J, Perry, J, 1971, 'Quadriceps function. An electromyographic study under isometric conditions', *Journal of Bone and Joint Surgery* 53A(4): 749

Marshall, J L, Gergis, F G, Zelko, R R, 1972, 'The biceps femoris tendon and its functional significance', *Journal of Bone and Joint Surgery* 54B: 1444

Martin, J A, Londeree, B R, 1979, 'EMG comparison of quadriceps femoris activity during knee extension and straight leg raises', *American Journal of Physical Medicine & Rehabilitation* 58: 57–69

Micheli, L, Slater, J, Woods, E, et al., 1986, 'Patella alta and the adolescent growth spurt', *Clinical Orthopaedics and Related Research* 213: 159–162

Newton, R A, 1982, 'Joint receptor contributions to reflexive and kinesthetic responses', *Physical Therapy* 62(1): 22–29

Radin, E L, Delamotte, F, Maquet, P, 1984, 'Role of the menisci in the distribution of stress in the knee', *Clinical Orthopaedics and Related Research* 185: 290–294

Renström, P, Johnson, R J, 1990, 'Anatomy and biomechanics of the menisci', *Clinical Orthopaedics and Related Research* 9(3): 523–538

Rowinski, M J, 1990, 'Afferent neurobiology of the joint', In: Gould, J A (ed.) *Orthopaedic and Sports Physical Therapy* pp. 49–63. C V Mosby Co, St Louis

Schultz, R, Miller, D, Kerr, C, Micheli, L, 1984, 'Mechanoreceptors in human cruciate ligaments', *Journal of Bone and Joint Surgery* 66A(7): 1072–1076

Shutte, M, Dabezies, E, Zimney, M, Happel, L, 1987, 'Neural anatomy of the human anterior cruciate ligament', *Journal of Bone and Joint Surgery* 69A(2): 243–247

Signorile, J F, Karsik, D, Perry, A, Robertson, B, Williams, R, Lowensteyn, I, Digel, S, Caruso, J, LeBlanc, W G, 1995, 'The effect of knee and foot position on the electromyographical activity of the superficial quadriceps', *Journal of Orthopaedic & Sports Physical Therapy* 22(1): 2–9

Skinner, H B, Wyatt, M P, Hodgdon, D W, Conard, D W, Barrack, R L, 1986, 'Effect of fatigue on joint position sense of the knee', *Journal of Orthopaedic Research* 4: 112–118

Tipton, C M, Matthes, R D, Maynard, J A, 1975, 'The influence of physical activity on ligaments and tendons', *Medicine and Science in Sports and Exercise* 7: 165–175

Warren, L F, Marshall, J L, 1979, 'The supporting structures and layers on the medial side of the knee: an anatomical analysis', *Journal of Bone and Joint Surgery* 61A: 56

Williams, P L, Bannister, L H, Berry, M M, Collins, P, Dyson, M, Dussek, J E, Ferguson, M W J, 1995, *Gray's Anatomy*, Churchill Livingstone, New York, Edinburgh, London, Tokyo, Madrid, Melbourne, 38th Edn

Knee pain and other symptoms

Amadio, P C, 1988, 'Pain dysfunction syndromes', *Journal of Bone and Joint Surgery* 70A: 944–949

Barrett, J, 1995, 'Reflex Sympathetic Dystrophy. Recognizing a cause of chronic pain', *Physician and Sportsmedicine* 23(4): 51–58

Brostoff, J, Challacombe, S J (eds), 1987, *Food Allergy and Intolerance*, Baillière Tindall, London

Brostoff, J, Gamlin, L, 1989, *The Complete Guide to Food Allergy and Intolerance*, Bloomsbury Publishing, London

Campa, J A, Broadnax, W, Broderick, J, et al., 1991, 'Neuropathic and sympathetically maintained pain complicating trauma or surgery to the knee', *Neurology (Suppl. 1)* 41: 165

Cooper, D E, DeLee, J C, Ramamurthy, S, 1989, 'Reflex Sympathetic Dystrophy of the knee. Treatment using continuous epidural anesthesia', *Journal of Bone and Joint Surgery* 71A: 365–369

Cooper, J, 1991, 'Food intolerance and joint symptoms – historical review and present-day application', *Physiotherapy* 77(12): 847–858

Davidoff, G, Werner, R, Cremer, S, et al., 1989, 'Predictive values of the three-phase Technetium bone scan in diagnosis of Reflex Sympathetic Dystrophy Syndrome', *Archives of Physical Medicine & Rehabilitation* 70(2): 135–137

Denman, A M, Mitchell, B, Ansell, B, 1983, 'Joint complaints and food allergic disorders', *Annals of Allergy* 51: 260–263

Fahrer, H, Rentsch, H U, Gerber, N J, Beyeler, C, Hess, C W, Grunig, B, 1988, 'Knee effusion and reflex inhibition of the quadriceps', *Journal of Bone and Joint Surgery* 70B: 635–638

Genant, H K, Kozin, F, Bekerman, C, et al., 1975, 'The Reflex Sympathetic Dystrophy Syndrome: a comprehensive analysis using fine-detail radiography, photon absorptiometry, and bone and joint scintigraphy', *Radiology* 117(1): 21–32

Johnson, M I, 1997, 'The physiology of the sensory dimensions of clinical pain', *Physiotherapy* 83(10): 526–536

Katz, M M, Hungerford, D S, 1987, 'Reflex Sympathetic Dystrophy affecting the knee', *Journal of Bone and Joint Surgery* 69B: 797–803

Kozin, F, Ryan, L M, Carrera, G F, et al., 1981, 'The Reflex Sympathetic Dystrophy Syndrome (RSDS): III scintigraphic studies, further evidence for the therapeutic efficacy of systemic corticosteroids, and proposed diagnostic criteria', *American Journal of Medicine* 70(1): 23–30

Lynch, M E, 1992, 'Psychological aspects of Reflex Sympathetic Dystrophy: a review of the adult and pediatric literature', *Pain* 49(3): 337–347

Marks, R, 1992, 'Peripheral articular mechanisms in pain production in osteo-arthritis', *Australian Journal of Physiotherapy* 38: 289–298

Merrit, J L, 1989, 'Soft tissue mechanisms of pain in osteoarthritis', *Seminars in Arthritis and Rheumatism, Suppl. 12* 18: 51–56

O'Brien, S J, Ngeow, J, Gibney, M A, Warren, R F, Fealy, S, 1996, 'Reflex Sympathetic Dystrophy of the knee: causes, diagnosis and treatment', *American Journal of Sports Medicine* 23(6): 655–659

Ogilvie-Harris, D J, Roscoe, M, 1987, 'Reflex Sympathetic Dystrophy of the knee', *Journal of Bone and Joint Surgery* 69B: 804–806

Schutzer, S F, Gossling, H R, 1984, 'The treatment of Reflex Sympathetic Dystrophy Syndrome', *Journal of Bone and Joint Surgery* 66A(4): 625–629

Schwartzman, R J, McLellan, T L, 1987, 'Reflex Sympathetic Dystrophy: a review', *Archives of Neurology* 44: 555–561

Seale, K S, 1989, 'Reflex Sympathetic Dystrophy of the lower extremity', *Clinical Orthopaedics and Related Research* 243: 80–85

Spencer, J, Hayes, K C, Alexander, I J, 1984, 'Knee joint effusion and quadriceps muscle inhibition in man', *Archives of Physical Medicine and Rehabilitation* 65: 171

Tietjen, R, 1986, 'Reflex Sympathetic Dystrophy of the knee', *Clinical Orthopaedics and Related Research* 209: 234–243

Waldman, S D, Waldman, K A, 1992, 'Reflex Sympathetic Dystrophy of the knee', *Journal of Pain and Symptom Management* 7: 243–245

Wall, P D, Melzack, R, 1994, *Textbook of Pain*, Churchill Livingstone, New York, Edinburgh, London, Melbourne, Tokyo, 3rd Edn

Zimmerman, M, 1989, 'Pain mechanisms and mediators in osteo-arthritis', *Seminars in Arthritis and Rheumatism, Suppl 2* 18: 22–29

Diagnosis and assessment

Bennett, G B, Stauber, W T, 1986, 'Evaluation and treatment of anterior knee pain using eccentric exercise', *Medicine and Science in Sports and Exercise* 18: 5

Chen, W-C, Wu, J J, Chang, C-Y, et al., 1987, 'Computed tomography of a meniscal cyst', *Orthopedics* 10: 1569–1572

Davies, G J, Larsen, R, 1978, 'Examining the knee', *Physician and Sportsmedicine* 6(4): 49

Davies, G J, Malone, T, Bassett, P H, 1980, 'Knee examination', *Physical Therapy* 60(12): 17

Ehman, R L, Berquist, T H, 1986, 'Magnetic resonance imaging of musculoskeletal trauma', *Radiological Clinics of North America* 24: 291–297

Frisch, H, 1994, *Systematic Musculoskeletal Examination*, Springer-Verlag, Heidelberg, 5th Edn

Hughston, J C, Norwood, L A, 1980, 'The posterolateral drawer test and external rotation recurvatum test for posterolateral rotatory instability of the knee', *Clinical Orthopaedics and Related Research* 147: 82

Maffulli, N, Regine, R, Carrillo, F, Minelli, S, Beaconsfield, T, 1992, 'Ultrasonographic scan in knee pain in athletes', *British Journal of Sports Medicine* 26(2): 93–96

Magee, D J, 1997, *Orthopedic Physical Assessment*, W B Saunders, Philadelphia, 3rd Edn

McLoughlin, R F, Raber, E L, Vellet, A D, Wiley, J P, Bray, R C, 1995, 'Patellar tendinitis: MR imaging features, with suggested pathogenesis and proposed classification', *Radiology* 197(3): 843–848

Noyes, F R, Barber, S, Mooar, L, 1989, 'A rationale for assessing sports activity levels and limitations in knee disorders', *Clinical Orthopaedics and Related Research* 246: 238–249

Noyes, F R, Grood, E S, Butler, D L, et al., 1980, 'Clinical laxity tests and functional stability of the knee: biomechanical concepts', *Clinical Orthopaedics and Related Research* 146: 84

Slocum, D B, James, S L, Larson, R L, et al., 1976, 'Clinical test for anterolateral rotatory instability of the knee', *Clinical Orthopaedics and Related Research* 118: 63

Slocum, D B, Larson, R L, 1968, 'Rotary instability of the knee, its pathogenesis and a clinical test to demonstrate its presence', *Journal of Bone and Joint Surgery* 50A: 211

Stickland, A, 1984, 'Examination of the knee joint', *Physiotherapy* 70(4): 144–150

Young, A, Hughes, I, Russell, P, Parker, M J, Nichols, P J R, 1980, 'Measurement of quadriceps muscle wasting by ultrasonography', *Rheumatology and Rehabilitation* 19: 141–148

Knee injuries – general

Beck, C, Drez, D, Young, J, 1986, 'Instrumented testing of functional knee braces', *American Journal of Sports Medicine* 14: 253–256

Berry, G A L, 1989, 'Assessment and treatment of knee injuries with particular attention to the hamstring muscles and joint swelling', *Physiotherapy* 75(1): 690–693

Coutts, F, Hewetson, D, Matthews, J, 1989, 'Continuous passive motion of the knee joint: use at the Royal National Orthopaedic Hospital, Stanmore', *Physiotherapy* 75(7): 427–431

Greenfield, B H, 1993, *Rehabilitation of the Knee: A Problem-Solving Approach*, F A Davis Company, Philadelphia

Helfet, A J, 1974, *Disorders of the Knee*, J B Lippincott, Philadelphia

Insall, J N (ed.), 1993, *Surgery of the Knee*, Churchill Livingstone, New York, Edinburgh, London, Melbourne, Tokyo, 2nd Edn

Kaeding, C C, Sanko, W A, Fischer, R A, 1995, 'Myositis ossificans: minimizing down-time', *Physician and Sportsmedicine* 23(2): 77–82

Mangine, R E, 1995, *Clinics in Physical Therapy: Physical Therapy of the Knee*, Churchill Livingstone, New York, Edinburgh, London, Melbourne, Tokyo, 2nd Edn

Munzinger, U, Ruckstuhl, J, Scherner, H, et al., 1981, 'Internal derangement of the knee due to pathologic synovial folds: the mediopatellar plica syndrome', *Clinical Orthopaedics and Related Research* 155: 59–64

Smillie, I S, 1978, *Injuries of the Knee Joint*, Churchill Livingstone, London and New York, 5th Edn

Smillie, I S, 1980, *Diseases of the Knee Joint*, Churchill Livingstone, Edinburgh, London, New York, 2nd Edn

Steiner, M E, 1987, 'Hypermobility and knee injuries', *Physician and Sportsmedicine* 15: 159–165

Zarins, B, Nemeth, V A, 1983, 'Acute knee injuries in athletes', *Clinics in Sports Medicine* 2: 149–166

Knee problems in children and adolescents

Anderson, S J, 1991, 'Overuse knee injuries in young athletes', *Physician and Sportsmedicine* 19(12): 69–80

Dinham, J M, 1975, 'Popliteal cysts in children: the case against surgery', *Journal of Bone and Joint Surgery* 57B: 69

Kennedy, J (ed.), 1979, *The Injured Adolescent Knee*, Williams and Wilkins, Baltimore, Maryland

Macnicol, M F, 1986, *The Problem Knee. Diagnosis and Management in the Younger Patient*, William Heinemann Medical Books, London

Mital, M A, Hayden, J, 1979, 'Pain in the knee in children: the medial plica shelf syndrome', *Orthopaedic Clinics of North America* 10(3): 713–722

Nisonson, B, 1989, 'Acute hemarthrosis of the adolescent knee', *Physician and Sportsmedicine* 17(4): 75–87

Scoles, P V, 1988, *Pediatric Orthopedics in Clinical Practice*, Year Book Medical Publishers Inc, Chicago, 2nd Edn

Singer, K, Henry, J, 1985, 'Knee problems in children and adolescents', *Clinics in Sports Medicine* 4: 385–397

Smith, A D, Tao, S S, 1995, 'Knee injuries in young athletes', *Clinics in Sports Medicine* 14(3): 629–650

Steiner, M E, Grana, W A, 1988, 'The young athlete's knee: recent advances', *Clinics in Sports Medicine* 7(3): 527–546

Kneecap pain syndrome

Beckman, M, Craig, R, Lehman, R C, 1989, 'Rehabilitation of patellofemoral dysfunction in the athlete', *Clinics in Sports Medicine* 8(4): 841–860

Bennett, J G, Stauber, W T, 1986, 'Evaluation and treatment of anterior knee pain using eccentric exercise', *Medicine and Science in Sports and Exercise* 18(5): 526–530

Bentley, G, Dowd, G, 1984, 'Current concepts of etiology and treatment of chondromalacia patella', *Clinical Orthopaedics and Related Research* 189: 209–228

Bockrath, K, Wooden, C, Worrell, T, Ingersoll, C D, Farr, J, 1993, 'Effects of patella taping on patella position and perceived pain', *Medicine and Science in Sports and Exercise* 989–992

Boucher, J P, Hodgdon, J A, 1993, 'Anatomical, mechanical, and functional factors in patello-femoral pain syndrome', *Chiropractic Sports Medicine* 7(1): 1–5

Boucher, J P, King, M A, Lefevre, R, Pépin, A, 1992, 'Quadriceps femoris muscle activity in patellofemoral pain syndrome', *American Journal of Sports Medicine* 20(5): 527–532

Brunet, M E, Stewart, G W, 1989, 'Patellofemoral rehabilitation', *Clinics in Sports Medicine* 8(2): 319–329

Callaghan, M J, Oldham, J A, 1996, 'The role of quadriceps exercise in the treatment of patellofemoral pain syndrome', *Sports Medicine* 21(5): 384–391

Cerny, K, 1995, 'Vastus medialis oblique/vastus lateralis muscle activity ratios for selected exercises in persons with and without patellofemoral pain syndrome', *Physical Therapy* 75(8): 672–683

Chesworth, B M, Culham, E G, Tata, G E, Peat, M, 1989, 'Validation of outcome measures in patients with patellofemoral syndrome', *Journal of Orthopaedic and Sports Physical Therapy* 12: 302–308

Crocker, B, Stauber, W, 1989, 'Objective analysis of quadriceps force during bracing of the patellae: a preliminary study', *Australian Journal of Science and Medicine in Sport* 25–28

Doucette, S A, Goble, E M, 1992, 'The effect of exercise on patellar tracking in lateral patellar compression syndrome', *American Journal of Sports Medicine* 20: 434–440

Dvir, Z, Shklar, A, Halperin, N, Robinson, D, Weissman, I, Ben-Shoshan, I, 1990, 'Concentric and eccentric torque variations of the quadriceps femoris in patellofemoral pain syndrome', *Clinical Biomechanics* 5: 68–72

Eisele, S A, 1991, 'A precise approach to anterior knee pain', *Physician and Sportsmedicine* 19(6): 127–139

Eng, J J, Pierrynowski, M R, 1993, 'Evaluation of soft foot orthotics in the treatment of patellofemoral pain syndrome', *Physical Therapy* 73(2): 62–68

Evans, I L, Paulos, L E, 1992, 'Complications of patellofemoral joint surgery', *Orthopaedic Clinics of North America* 23: 697–707

Felder, C R, Leeson, M A, 1990, *Patellofemoral Pain Syndrome: the Use of Electro-myographic Biofeedback for Training the Vastus Medialis Obliquus in Patients with Patellofemoral Pain*, Electromyography Applications in Physical Therapy, Thought Technology Ltd, USA

Flynn, T W, Soutas-Little, R W, 1995, 'Patellofemoral joint compressive forces in forward and backward running', *Journal of Orthopaedic & Sports and Physical Therapy* 21(5): 277–282

Ford, D H, Post, W R, 1997, 'Open or arthroscopic lateral release: indications, techniques and rehabilitation', *Arthroscopic Surgery of the Knee* 16(1): 29–49

Fulkerson, J P, Hungerford, D S, 1990, *Disorders of the Patellofemoral Joint*, Williams and Wilkins, Baltimore, Maryland

Gaffney, K, Fricker, P, Dwyer, T, Barrett, E, Skibinski, K, Coutts, R, 1992, 'Patellofemoral joint pain: a comparison of two treatment programmes', *Excel* 8: 179–189

Galanty, H L, Matthews, C, Hergenroeder, A C, 1994, 'Anterior knee pain in adolescents', *Clinical Journal of Sports Medicine* 4: 176–181

Galea, A M, Albers, J M, 1994, 'Patellofemoral pain: beyond empirical diagnosis', *Physician and Sportsmedicine* 22(4): 48–58

Goldberg, B, 1991, 'Chronic anterior knee pain in the adolescent', *Pediatric Annals* 20(4): 186–193

Grana, W A, Hinkley, B, Hollingsworth, S, 1984, 'Arthroscopic evaluation and treatment of patellar malalignment', *Clinical Orthopaedics and Related Research* 186: 122–128

Gulling, L K, Lephart, S M, Stone, D A, Irrgang, J J, Pincivero, D M, 1996, 'The effects of patellar bracing on quadriceps EMG activity during isokinetic exercise', *Isokinetics and Exercise Science* 6: 133–138

Harrington, L, Payton, C J, 1997, 'Effects of corrective taping of the patella on patients with patellofemoral pain', *Physiotherapy* 83(11): 566–572

Hilyard, A, 1990, 'Recent developments in the management of patellofemoral pain: the McConnell Programme', *Physiotherapy* 76(9): 559–565

Hughston, J C, Deese, M, 1988, 'Medial subluxation of the patella as a complication of lateral retinacular release', *American Journal of Sports Medicine* 16(4): 383–388

Ingersoll, C D, Knight, K L, 1991, 'Patellar location changes following EMG biofeedback or progressive resistance exercises', *Medicine and Science in Sports and Exercise* 23(10): 1122–1127

Insall, J, 1979, 'Chondromalacia patellae: patellar malalignment syndrome', *Orthopaedic Clinics of North America* 10: 117–127

Johnson, D, Thurston P, Ashcroft P, 1977, 'The Russian technique of faradism in the treatment of chondromalacia patellae', *Physiotherapy Canada* 29: 2–4

Kannus, P, Nittymäki, S, 1994, 'Which factors predict outcome in the nonoperative treatment of patellofemoral pain syndrome? A prospective follow-up study', *Medicine and Science in Sport and Exercise* 289–296

Karlsson, J, Thomeé, R, Swärd, L, 1996, 'Eleven-year follow-up of patello-femoral pain syndrome', *Clinical Journal of Sports Medicine* 6(1): 22–24

Kettlecamp, D B, 1981, 'Management of patellar malalignment', *Journal of Bone and Joint Surgery* 63B: 1344–1347

Kowall, M G, Kolk, G, Nuber, G W, Cassisi, J E, Stern, S H, 1996, 'Patellar taping in the treatment of patellofemoral pain, *American Journal of Sports Medicine* 24(1): 61–66

LaBrier, K, O'Neill, D B, 1993, 'Patellofemoral stress syndrome', *Sports Medicine* 16(6): 449–459

Larsen, B, Andreasen, E, Urfer, A, Mickelsen, M R, Newhouse, K E, 1996, 'Patellar taping: a radiographic examination of the medial glide technique', *American Journal of Sports Medicine* 23(4): 465–471

LeVeau, B, Rogers, C, 1980, 'Selective training of the vastus medialis muscle using EMG biofeedback', *Physiotherapy* 60(11): 1410–1415

Macintyre, D, Wessel, J, 1988, 'Knee muscle torques in patellofemoral pain syndrome', *Physiotherapy Canada* 40(1): 20–23

Mäenpää, H, Lehto M U K, 1995, 'Surgery in acute patellar dislocation – evaluation of the effect of injury mechanism and family occurrence on the outcome of treatment', *British Journal of Sports Medicine* 29(4): 239–241

Malek, M M, Fanelli, G C, 1991, 'Patellofemoral pain: an arthroscopic perspective', *Clinics in Sports Medicine* 10(3): 549–567

Malek, M M, Mangine, R E, 1981, 'Patellofemoral pain syndromes: a comprehensive and conservative approach', *Journal of Orthopaedic & Sports Physical Therapy* 2: 108–116

McConnell, J, 1986, 'The management of chondromalacia patellae: a long term solution', *Australian Journal of Physiotherapy* 32(4): 215–223

McConnell, J, 1996, 'Management of patellofemoral problems', *Manual Therapy* 1: 60–66

O'Neill, D B, Micheli, L J, Warner, J P, 1992, 'Patellofemoral stress: a prospective analysis of exercise treatment in adolescents and adults', *American Journal of Sports Medicine* 20(2): 151–156

Outerbridge, R E, 1961, 'The etiology of chondromalacia patellae', *Journal of Bone and Joint Surgery* 43B: 752–757

Pickett, J C, Radin, E L, 1983, *Chondromalacia of the Patella*, Williams and Wilkins, Baltimore, Maryland

Puniello, M S, 1996, 'Iliotibial band tightness and medial patellar glide in patients with patellofemoral dysfunction', *Journal of Orthopaedic & Sports Physical Therapy* 17(3): 144–148

Reynolds, L, Levin, T A, Medeiros, J M, Adler, N S, Hallum, A, 1983, 'EMG activity of the vastus medialis oblique and the vastus lateralis in their role in patellar alignment', *American Journal of Physical Medicine & Rehabilitation* 62: 61–70

Scaringe, J, 1994, 'Patellofemoral pain syndrome', *Chiropractic Sports Medicine* 8(4): 161–162

Selfe, J, Gillard, D L, Marshall, S C, 1996, 'Patello-femoral pain: is the A-angle a clinically useful measurement?' *Physiotherapy* 82(5): 324–330

Shelton, G L, 1992, 'Conservative management of patellofemoral dysfunction', *Primary Care* 19(2): 331–350

Shelton, G L, Thigpen, L K, 1991, 'Rehabilitation of patellofemoral dysfunction: a review of literature', *Journal of Orthopaedic & Sports Physical Therapy* 14(6): 243–248

Steinkamp, L A, Dillingham, M F, Markel, M D, Hill, J A, Kaufman, K R, 1993, 'Biomechanical considerations in patellofemoral joint rehabilitation', *American Journal of Sports Medicine* 21(3): 438–444

Stiene, H A, Brosky, T, Reinking, M F, Nyland, J, Mason, M B, 1996, 'A comparison of closed kinetic chain and isokinetic joint isolation exercise in patients with patellofemoral dysfunction', *Journal of Orthopaedic and Sports Physical Therapy* 24(3): 136–141

Thomeé, R, Grimby, G, Svantesson, U, Österberg, U, 1996, 'Quadriceps muscle performance in sitting and standing in young women with patellofemoral pain syndrome and young healthy women', *Scandinavian Journal of Medicine and Science in Sports* 6: 233–241

Thomeé, R, Renström, P, Karlsson, J, Grimby, G, 1995, 'Patellofemoral pain syndrome in young women', *Scandinavian Journal of Medicine and Science in Sports* 5: 237–244

Tria, A J, Palumbo, R C, 1992, 'Conservative care for patellofemoral pain', *Orthopaedic Clinics of North America* 23: 545–553

Wild, J, Franklin, R, Woods, G, 1982, 'Patellar pain and quadriceps rehabilitation', *American Journal of Sports Medicine* 10: 12–15

Williams, J G P, Street, M, 1976, 'Sequential faradism in quadriceps rehabilitation', *Physiotherapy* 62(8): 252–254

Wilson, T, 1990, 'Anterior knee pain: a new technique for examination and treatment', *Physiotherapy* 76(7): 371–376

Wise, H H, Fiebert, I M, Kates, J L, 1984, 'EMG biofeedback as treatment for patello-femoral pain syndrome', *Journal of Orthopaedic & Sports Physical Therapy* 6: 95–103

Woodall, W, Welsh, J, 1990, 'A biomechanical basis for rehabilitation programs involving the patellofemoral joint', *Journal of Orthopaedic & Sports Physical Therapy* 11: 535–542

Zappala, F G, Taffel, C B, 1992, 'Rehabilitation of patellofemoral joint disorders', *Orthopaedic Clinics of North America* 23: 555–565

Bone injuries

Antich, T J, Brewster, C E, 1985, 'Osgood-Schlatter's disease. Review of literature and physical therapy management', *Journal of Orthopaedic & Sports Physical Therapy* 7: 5–10

Beovich, R, Fricker, P A, 1988, 'Osgood-Schlatter's disease. A review of the literature and an Australian series', *Australian Journal of Science and Medicine in Sport* 20(4): 11–13

Bertin, K, Goble, E, 1983, 'Ligament injuries associated with physeal fractures about the knee', *Clinical Orthopaedics and Related Research* 177: 188–195

Bourne, M K, Bianco, A J, 1990, 'Bipartite patella in the adolescent: results of surgical excision', *Journal of Pediatric Orthopedics* 10: 69–73

Bowers, K D, 1981, 'Patellar tendon avulsion as a complication of Osgood-Schlatter's disease', *American Journal of Sports Medicine* 9: 356–359

Cahill, B, 1985, 'Treatment of juvenile osteochondritis dissecans and osteochondritis dissecans of the knee', *Clinics in Sports Medicine* 4: 367–384

Clanton, T O, DeLee, J C, 1982, 'Osteochondritis dissecans: history pathophysiology and current treatment concepts', *Clinical Orthopaedics and Related Research* 167: 50–64

Devas, M, 1975, *Stress Fractures*, Churchill Livingstone, Edinburgh, London, New York

Douglas, G, Rand, M, 1981, 'The role of trauma in the pathogenesis of the osteochondroses', *Clinical Orthopaedics and Related Research* 158: 28–32

Federico, D J, Lynch, J K, Jokl, P, 1990, 'Osteochondritis dissecans of the knee: a historical review of the etiology and treatment', *Arthroscopy* 6(3): 190–197

Garth, W P, Pomphrey, M, Merrill, K, 1996, 'Functional treatment of patellar dislocation in an athletic population', *American Journal of Sports Medicine* 24(6): 785–791

Gill, J, Chakrabarti, H, Becker, S, 1983, 'Fractures of the proximal tibial epiphysis', *Injury* 14: 324–331

Hensal, F, Nelson, T, Pavlow, H, Torg, J, 1983, 'Bilateral patella fractures from indirect trauma', *Clinical Orthopaedics and Related Research* 178: 207–209

Holmes, C A, Bach, B R, 1995, 'Knee dislocations: immediate and definitive care', *Physician and Sportsmedicine* 23(11): 69–82

Hughston, J, Hergenroeder, P, Courtenay, B, 1984, 'Osteochondritis dissecans of the femoral condyles', *Journal of Bone and Joint Surgery* 66A: 1340–1348

Hutchinson, M R, Lloyd Ireland, M, 1995, 'Patella dislocation: recognizing the injury and its complications', *Physician and Sportsmedicine* 23(10): 53–60

Kobayashi, Y, Sukawa, T, Nagano, J, et al., 1990, 'Surgical treatment of the painful bipartite patellae', *The Knee* 16: 46–49

Kujala, U, Kvist, M, Heinonen, O, 1985, 'Osgood-Schlatter's disease in adolescent athletes', *American Journal of Sports Medicine* 13: 236–241

Kurzweil, P R, Zambetti, G J, Hamilton, W G, 1988, 'Osteochondritis dissecans in the lateral patellofemoral groove', *American Journal of Sports Medicine* 16(3): 308–310

Larson, E, Lauridsen, F, 1982, 'Conservative treatment of patellar dislocation', *Clinical Orthopaedics and Related Research* 171: 131

Letts, R M, 1994, *Management of Pediatric Fractures*, Churchill Livingstone, New York, Edinburgh, London, Melbourne, Tokyo

Mäenpää, H, Lehto, M U K, 1995, 'Surgery in acute patellar dislocation – evaluation of the effect of injury mechanism and family occurrence on the outcome of treatment', *British Journal of Sports Medicine* 29(4): 239–241

Mbubaegbu, C E, 1994, 'Femoral osteochondral fracture – a non-contact injury in martial arts? A case report', *British Journal of Sports Medicine* 28(3): 203–205

McRae, R, 1994, *Practical Fracture Treatment*, Churchill Livingstone, New York, Edinburgh, London, Melbourne, Tokyo, 3rd Edn

Micheli, L J, 1987, 'The traction apophysitises', *Clinics in Sports Medicine* 6: 389–404

Mirbey, J, Besancenot, J, Chambers, R T, Durey, A, Vichard, P, 1988,

'Avulsion fractures of the tibial tuberosity in the adolescent athlete', *American Journal of Sports Medicine* 16(4): 336–340

Mori, Y, Okumo, H, Iketani, H, Kuroki, Y, 1996, 'Efficacy of lateral retinacular release for painful bipartite patella', *American Journal of Sports Medicine* 23(1): 13–18

Mubarak, S, Carroll, N, 1981, 'Juvenile osteochondritis dissecans of the knee', *Clinical Orthopaedics and Related Research* 157: 200–211

Obedian, R S, Grelsamer, R P, 1997, 'Osteochondritis dissecans of the distal femur and patella', *Clinics in Sports Medicine* 16(1): 157–174

Ogden, J A, McCarthy, S M, Jokl, P, 1984, 'The painful bipartite patella', *Journal of Pediatric Orthopedics* 2(3): 263–269

Ogden, J A, Southwick, W O, 1976, 'Osgood-Schlatter's disease and tibial tuberosity development', *Clinical Orthopaedics and Related Research* 116: 180–189

Ogden, J A, Tross, R B, Murphy, M J, 1980, 'Fractures of the tibial tuberosity in adolescents', *Journal of Bone and Joint Surgery* 62A: 205–215

Omer, G E, 1981, 'Primary articular osteochondroses', *Clinical Orthopaedics and Related Research* 158: 33–40

Orava, S, Taimela, S, Karpakka, J, Hulkko, A, Kujala, U, 1996, 'Diagnosis and treatment of stress fracture of the patella in athletes', *Knee Surgery, Sports Traumatology, Arthroscopy* 4(4): 206–211

Orava, S, Virtanen, K, 1982, 'Osteochondroses in athletes', *British Journal of Sports Medicine* 16(3): 161–168

Outerbridge, R E, 1983, 'Osteochondritis dissecans of the posterior femoral condyle', *Clinical Orthopaedics and Related Research* 175: 121–129

Pietu, G, Hauet, P, 1995, 'Stress fracture of the patella', *Acta Orthopaedica Scandinavica* 66(5): 481–482

Sailors, M E, 1994, 'Recognition and treatment of osteochondritis dissecans of the femoral condyles', *Journal of Athletic Training* 29(4): 302, 304, 306

Sallay, P I, Poggi, J, Speer, K P, Garrett, W E, 1996, 'Acute dislocation of the patella: a correlative pathoanatomic study', *American Journal of Sports Medicine* 24(1): 52–60

Shelton, W R, Canale, S T, 1979, 'Fractures of the tibia through the proximal epiphyseal cartilage', *Journal of Bone and Joint Surgery* 61A: 167–173

Vince, K G, 1987, 'Osteochondritis dissecans of the knee', *Orthopaedic Clinics of North America* 18(4): 555–576

Walter, N, Wolf, M, 1977, 'Stress fractures in young athletes', *American Journal of Sports Medicine* 5: 165–170

Weaver, J K, 1977, 'Bipartite patellae as a cause of disability in the athlete', *American Journal of Sports Medicine* 5(4): 137–143

Osteoarthritis and degenerative arthritis

Aubin, M, Marks, R, 1995, 'The efficacy of short-term treatment with transcutaneous electrical nerve stimulation for osteo-arthritic knee pain', *Physiotherapy* 81(11): 669–675

Casscells, S W, 1985, 'The torn meniscus, the torn anterior cruciate ligament, and their relationship to degenerative joint disease', *Arthroscopy* 1: 28

Gose, J, 1987, 'Continuous passive motion in the post-operative treatment of patients with total knee replacement', *Physical Therapy* 67(1): 39–42

Graham, G P, Fairclough, J A, 1988, 'Early osteoarthritis in young sportsmen with severe anterolateral instability of the knee', *Injury* 19(4): 247–248

Harms, M, Engstrom, B, 1991, 'Continuous passive motion as an adjunct to treatment in the physiotherapy management of the total knee arthroplasty patient', *Physiotherapy* 77(4): 301–307

Kannus, P, Järvinen, M, 1988, 'Osteo-arthrosis in a knee joint due to chronic post-traumatic insufficiency of the medial collateral ligament: nine-year follow-up', *Clinical Rheumatology* 7: 200–207

Marks, R, Cantin, D, 1997, 'Symptomatic osteo-arthritis of the knee: the efficacy of physiotherapy', *Physiotherapy* 83(6): 306–312

Messier, S P, Loeser, R F, Hoover, J L, Semble, E L, 1992, 'Osteo-arthritis of the knee: effects on gait, strength and flexibility', *Archives of Physical Medicine and Rehabilitation* 73: 29–36

Stockwell, R A, 1991, 'Cartilage failure in osteo-arthritis: relevance of normal structure and function: a review', *Clinical Anatomy* 4: 161–191

Cartilage injuries

DeHaven, K E, 1990, 'Decision-making factors in the treatment of meniscus lesions', *Clinics in Orthopaedics and Related Research* 252: 49

DeHaven, K E, Bronstein, R D, 1997, 'Arthroscopic medial meniscal repair in the athlete', *Clinics in Sports Medicine* 16(1): 69–86

Dickhaut, S, DeLee, J, 1982, 'The discoid lateral meniscus syndrome', *Journal of Bone and Joint Surgery* 64A: 1068–1073

Fahmy, N R M, Williams, E A, Noble, J, 1983, 'Meniscal pathology and osteoarthritis of the knee', *Journal of Bone and Joint Surgery* 65B: 24

Levy, M, Torzilli, P A, Warren, R F, 1982, 'The effect of medial meniscectomy on anterior/posterior motion of the knee', *Journal of Bone and Joint Surgery* 64A: 883

McLaughlin et al., 1994, 'Rehabilitation after meniscus repair', *Journal of Orthopaedic Research* 17: 463

Manzione, M, Pizzutillo, P, Peoples, A, 1983, 'Meniscectomy in children: a long-term follow-up study', *American Journal of Sports Medicine* 11: 111–115

Matthews, P, St Pierre, D M M, 1996, 'Recovery of muscle strength following arthroscopic meniscectomy', *Medicine and Sport Science* 23(1): 18–26

Northmore-Ball, M D, Dandy, D J, Jackson, R W, 1983, 'Arthroscopic, open partial, and total meniscectomy: a comparative study', *Journal of Bone and Joint Surgery* 65B: 400

Raskas, D, Lehman, R C, 1988, 'Meniscal injuries in athletes: pinpointing the diagnosis', *Journal of Musculoskeletal Medicine* 5: 18

Shakespeare, D T, Stokes, M, Sherman, K P, Young, A, 1983, 'The effect of knee flexion on quadriceps inhibition after meniscectomy', *Clinical Science* 65: 64–65

Shelbourne, K D, Patel, D V, Adsit, W S, Potter, D A, 1996, 'Rehabilitation after meniscal repair', *Clinics in Sports Medicine* 15(3): 595–612

Stone, R G, Frewin, P R, Gonzales, S, 1990, 'Long-term assessment of arthroscopic meniscus repair: a two-to-six-year follow-up study', *Arthroscopy* 6: 73

Cruciate ligament injuries

Anderson, A F, Lipscomb, A B, 1989, 'Analysis of rehabilitation techniques after anterior cruciate reconstruction', *American Journal of Sports Medicine* 17(2): 154–160

Barrack, R, Bruckner, J, Kneisl, J, Inman, W, Alexander, H, 1990, 'The outcome of non-operatively treated complete tears of the anterior cruciate ligament in active young adults', *Clinical Orthopaedics and Related Research* 259: 192–199

Barrack, R L, Skinner, H B, Buckley, S L, 1989, 'Proprioception in the anterior cruciate deficient knee', *Physician and Sportsmedicine* 11(6): 1–6

Blackburn, T A, 1992, 'Rehabilitation of anterior instability of the knee', *Journal of Sport Rehabilitation* 1: 132–145

Blair, D F, Wills, R P, 1991, 'Rapid rehabilitation following anterior cruciate ligament reconstruction', *Athletic Trainer* 26: 32–43

Bonamo, J, Fay, C, Firestone, T, 1990, 'The conservative treatment of the anterior cruciate deficient knee', *American Journal of Sports Medicine* 18(6): 618–623

Buseck, M S, Noyes, F, 1991, 'Arthroscopic evaluation of meniscal repairs after anterior cruciate ligament reconstruction and immediate motion', *American Journal of Sports Medicine* 19(5): 489–494

Carter, N D, Jenkinson, T R, Wilson, D, Jones, D W, Torode, A S, 1997, 'Joint position sense and rehabilitation in the anterior cruciate ligament deficient knee', *British Journal of Sports Medicine* 31: 209–212

Clark, P, MacDonald, P B, Sutherland, K, 1996, 'Analysis of proprioception in the posterior cruciate ligament-deficient knee', *Knee Surgery, Sports Traumatology, Arthroscopy* 4(4): 225–227

Draper, V, 1990, 'Electromyographic biofeedback and recovery of quadriceps femoris muscle function following anterior cruciate ligament reconstruction', *Physical Therapy* 70(1): 11–17

Feagin, J A (ed.), 1994, *The Crucial Ligaments: Diagnosis and Treatment of Ligamentous Injuries about the Knee*, Churchill Livingstone, New York, Edinburgh, London, Melbourne, Tokyo

Fu, F H, Woo, S L Y, Irrgang, J J, 1992, 'Current concepts for rehabilitation following anterior cruciate ligament reconstruction', *Journal of Orthopaedic & Sports Physical Therapy* 15: 270–278

Holmes, P F, James, S L, Larson, R L, Singer, K M, Jones, D L, 1991, 'Retrospective direct comparison of three intra-articular anterior cruciate ligament reconstructions', *American Journal of Sports Medicine* 19: 596–599

Kannus, P, 1988, 'Ratio of hamstring to quadriceps femoris muscles' strength in the anterior cruciate ligament insufficient knee. Relationship to long term recovery', *Physical Therapy* 6: 961–965

Lipscomb, P, Naderson, A, 1986, 'Tears of the anterior cruciate ligament in adolescents', *Journal of Bone and Joint Surgery* 68A: 19–28

MacDonald, P B, Hedden, D, Pacin, O, Sutherland, K, 1996, 'Proprioception in anterior cruciate ligament-deficient and reconstructed knees', *American Journal of Sports Medicine* 24(6): 774–778

Malone, T R, Garrett, W E, 1992, 'Commentary and historical perspective of anterior cruciate ligament rehabilitation', *Journal of Orthopaedic & Sports Physical Therapy* 15: 265–269

McCarroll, J R, Shelbourne, K D, Patel, D V, 1995, 'Anterior cruciate ligament injuries in young athletes: recommendations for treatment and rehabilitation', *Sports Medicine* 20(2): 117–127

Mizuta, H, Kubota, K, Shiraishi, M, Otsuka, Y, Nagamoto, N, Takagi, K, 1995, 'The conservative treatment of complete tears of the anterior cruciate ligament in skeletally immature patients', *Journal of Bone and Joint Surgery* 77(6): 890–894

Morrissey, M C, Brewster, C E, 1986, 'Hamstring weakness after surgery for anterior cruciate injury', *Journal of Orthopaedic & Sports Physical Therapy* 7: 310–313

Noyes, F R, Mangine, R E, Berber, S, 1987, 'Early knee motion after open and arthroscopic anterior ligament reconstruction', *American Journal of Sports Medicine* 15: 149–160

Seto, J, Brewster, C, Lombardo, S, Tibone, J, 1989, 'Rehabilitation of the knee after anterior cruciate ligament reconstruction', *Journal of Orthopaedic & Sports Physical Therapy* 11(1): 8–18

Shino, K, Horibe, S, Nakata, K, Maeda, A, Hamada, M, Nakamura, N,

1995, 'Conservative treatment of isolated injuries to the posterior cruciate ligament in athletes', *Journal of Bone and Joint Surgery* 77(6): 895–900

Suart, W M, Patrick, M A, Betts, H J, Murray, A, Pope, J A, 1988, 'Rehabilitation following Dacron graft reconstruction of the anterior cruciate ligament of the knee', *Physiotherapy* 74(10): 528–530

Tibone, J E, Antich, T J, 1988, 'A biomechanical analysis of the anterior cruciate ligament repair with the patellar tendon', *American Journal of Sports Medicine* 16: 332

Timm, K E, 1997, 'The clinical and cost-effectiveness of two different programmes for rehabilitation following ACL construction', *Journal of Orthopaedic & Sports Physical Therapy* 25(1): 43–48

Wilk, K E, Andrews, J R, 1992, 'Current concepts in the treatment of anterior cruciate ligament disruption', *Journal of Orthopaedic & Sports Physical Therapy* 15: 279–293

Zätterström, R, Fridén, T, Lindstrand, A, Moritz, U, 1994, 'The effect of physiotherapy on standing balance in chronic anterior cruciate ligament insufficiency', *American Journal of Sports Medicine* 22(4): 531–536

Ligament injuries

Engle, R P, 1991, *Knee Ligament Rehabilitation*, Churchill Livingstone, New York, Edinburgh, London, Melbourne, Tokyo

Hede, A, Hejgaard, N, Sandberg, H, Jacobsen, K, 1985, 'Sports injuries of the knee ligaments – a prospective stress radiographic study', *British Journal of Sports Medicine* 19(1): 8–10

Indelicato, P, 1983, 'Non-operative treatment of complete tears of the medial collateral ligament of the knee', *Journal of Bone and Joint Surgery* 65A: 323–329

Inoue, M, McGurk-Burleson, E, Hollis, J M, Wood, S L-Y, 1987, 'Treatment of the medial collateral ligament injury', *American Journal of Sports Medicine* 15: 15

Jenkins, D H R, 1985, *Ligament Injuries and their Treatment*, Chapman and Hall Medical, London

Kannus, P, Järvinen, M, 1987, 'Long-term prognosis of conservatively treated acute knee ligament injuries in competitive and spare time sportsmen', *International Journal of Sports Medicine* 8: 348–351

Kannus, P, Järvinen, M, 1991, 'Thigh muscle function after partial tear of the medial ligament compartment of the knee', *Medicine and Science in Sports and Exercise* 23(1): 4–9

Meislin, R J, 1996, 'Managing collateral ligament tears of the knee', *Physician and Sportsmedicine* 24(3): 67–74

Reider, B, 1996, 'Medial collateral ligament injuries in athletes', *Sports Medicine* 21(2): 147–156

Scott, W N (ed.), 1991, *Ligament and Extensor Mechanisms of the Knee: Diagnosis and Treatment*, C V Mosby Co, St Louis

Tria, A J, 1995, *Ligaments of the Knee*, Churchill Livingstone International, New York, Edinburgh, London, Melbourne, Tokyo

Woo, S L-Y, Ohno, K, Weaver, C M, Pomaybo, A S, Xerogeanes, J W, 1994, 'Non-operative treatment of knee ligament injuries', *Sports Exercise and Injury* 1: 2–13

Iliotibial tract (band) injuries

Aronen, J G, Chronister, R, Regan, K, Hensien, M A, 1993, 'Practical, conservative management of iliotibial band syndrome', *Physician and Sportsmedicine* 21(6): 59–69

Gose, J, Schweizer, P, 1989, 'Iliotibial band tightness', *Journal of Orthopaedic & Sports Physical Therapy* 10: 399–407

Lindenburg, G, Pinshaw, R, Noakes, T D, 1984, 'Iliotibial band friction syndrome in runners', *Physician and Sportsmedicine* 12: 118–130

Martens, M, Libbrecht, P, Burssens, A, 1989, 'Surgical treatment of the iliotibial band friction syndrome', *American Journal of Sports Medicine* 17(5): 651–654

Noble, C A, 1979, 'The treatment of iliotibial band friction syndrome', *British Journal of Sports Medicine* 13: 51–54

Noble, C A, 1980, 'Iliotibial band friction syndrome in runners', *American Journal of Sports Medicine* 8(4): 232–234

Noble, H B, Hajek, R, Porter, M, 1982, 'Diagnosis and treatment of iliotibial band tightness in runners', *Physician and Sportsmedicine* 10: 67–74

Orava, S, 1978, 'Iliotibial tract friction syndrome in athletes – an uncommon exertion syndrome on the lateral side of the knee', *British Journal of Sports Medicine* 12(2): 69–73

Renne, J W, 1975, 'The iliotibial band friction syndrome', *Journal of Bone and Joint Surgery* 57A: 1110–1111

Rouse, S J, 1996, 'The role of the iliotibial tract in patellofemoral pain and iliotibial band friction syndromes', *Physiotherapy* 82(3): 199–202

Schwellnus, M P, Mackintosh, L, Mee, J, 1992, 'Deep transverse frictions in the treatment of iliotibial band friction syndrome in athletes: a clinical trial', *Physiotherapy* 78(8): 564–568

Stanish, W D, Rabinovich, M, Curwin, K S, 1986, 'Eccentric exercise in chronic tendinitis', *Clinical Orthopaedics and Related Research* 208: 65–69

Sutker, A, Jackson, D, Pagliano, J, 1981, 'Iliotibial band friction syndrome in distance runners', *Physician and Sportsmedicine* 9: 69–73

Westers, B, Beaton, P, 1988, 'Iliotibial tract syndrome (case study)', *Physiotherapy* 74(12): 637

Patellar tendon problems

Blazina, M E, Kerlan, R K, Jobe, F W, Carter, V S, Carlson, R N, 1973, 'Jumper's knee', *Orthopaedic Clinics of North America* 4(3): 665–678

Colosimo, A J, Bassett, F H, 1990, 'Jumper's knee. Diagnosis and treatment', *Orthopaedic Review* 19(2): 139–149

Ferretti, A, 1986, 'Epidemiology of jumper's knee', *Sports Medicine* 3: 289–295

Jenson, K, DiFabio, R P, 1989, 'Evaluation of eccentric exercise in the treatment of patellar tendinitis', *Physical Therapy* 69: 211–216

Kibler, W B, 1997, 'Diagnosis, treatment and rehabilitation principles in complete tendon ruptures in sports', *Scandinavian Journal of Medicine and Science in Sports* 7: 119–129

King, J B, Perry, J D, Mourad, K, Kumar, S I, 1990, 'Lesions of the patellar ligament', *Journal of Bone and Joint Surgery* 72B: 46–48

Laseter, J T, Russel, J A, 1991, 'Anabolic steroid-induced tendon pathology: a review of the literature', *Medicine and Science in Sports and Exercise* 23: 1–3

Liow, R Y L, Tavares, S, 1995, 'Bilateral rupture of the quadriceps tendon associated with anabolic steroids', *British Journal of Sports Medicine* 29(2): 77–79

Martens, M, Wouters, P, Burssens, A, Mulier, J C, 1982, 'Patellar tendinitis: pathology and results of treatment', *Acta Orthopedica Scandinavica* 53: 445–450

Medlar, R C, Lyne, E D, 1978, 'Sinding-Larsen-Johansson disease: its etiology and natural history', *Journal of Bone and Joint Surgery* 60A: 1113–1116

Orava, S, Österback, L, Hurme, M, 1986, 'Surgical treatment of patellar tendon pain in athletes', *British Journal of Sports Medicine* 20(4): 167–169

Richards, D P, Ajemian, S V, Wiley, J P, Zernicke, R F, 1996, 'Knee joint mechanics predict patellar tendinitis in elite volleyball players', *American Journal of Sports Medicine* 24(5): 676–683

Roels, J, Martens, M, Mulier, J C, Burssens, A, 1978, 'Patellar tendinitis (jumper's knee)', *American Journal of Sports Medicine* 6: 362–368

Stanish, W D, Rabinovich, M, Curwin, K S, 1986, 'Eccentric exercise in chronic tendinitis', *Clinical Orthopaedics and Related Research* 208: 65–69

Torstensen, E T, Bray, R C, Wiley, J P, 1994, 'Patellar tendinitis: a review of current concepts and treatment', *Clinical Journal of Sports Medicine* 4: 77–82

Electrical muscle stimulation

Arvidsson, I, Arvidsson, H, Eriksson, E, Jansson, E, 1986, 'Prevention of quadriceps muscle wasting after immobilization: an evaluation of the effect of electrical stimulation', *Orthopedics* 9: 1519–1528

Bohannon, R W, 1983, 'Effect of electrical stimulation to the vastus medialis muscle in a patient with chronically dislocating patellae', *Physical Therapy* 63: 1445–1447

Boutelle, D, Smith, B, Malone, T, 1985, 'A strength study utilizing the Electrostim 180', *Journal of Orthopaedic & Sports Physical Therapy* 7: 50–53

Caggiano, E, Emrey, T, Shirley, S, Craik, R L, 1994, 'Effects of electrical stimulation or voluntary contraction for strengthening the quadriceps femoris muscle in an aged male population', *Journal of Orthopaedic & Sports Physical Therapy* 20(1): 22–28

Charman, R A, 1990, 'Bioelectricity and electrotherapy – towards a new paradigm?' *Physiotherapy* 76(9): 502–516

Convery, A, Racer, B, Rohland, R, Shannon, J, Sorg, J, 1994, 'The effects of electrical stimulation and electromyographic biofeedback on muscle performance output with training of the quadriceps femoris muscle', *Isokinetics and Exercise Science* 4(3): 122–127

Currier, D P, Mann, R, 1983, 'Muscular strength development by electrical stimulation in healthy individuals', *Physical Therapy* 63: 915–921

Currier, D P, Ray, J M, Nyland, J, Rooney, J G, Noteboom, J T, Kellogg, R, 1993, 'Effects of electrical and electromagnetic stimulation after anterior cruciate ligament reconstruction', *Journal of Orthopaedic & Sports Physical Therapy* 17(4): 177–184

Delitto, A, McKowen, J M, McCarthy, J A, Lehman, R C, Thomas, J A, Shively, R A, 1988, 'Electrically elicited co-contraction of thigh musculature after anterior cruciate ligament surgery', *Physical Therapy* 68: 45–50

Delitto, A, Snyder-Mackler, L, 1990, 'Two theories of muscle strength augmentation using percutaneous electrical stimulation', *Physical Therapy* 70: 158–164

Gauthier, J M, Thériault, R, Thériault, G, Gélinas, Y, Simoneau, J-A, 1992, 'Electrical stimulation-induced changes in skeletal muscle enzymes of men and women', *Medicine and Science in Sports and Exercise* 24: 1252–1256

Gibson, J N A, Morrison, W L, Scrimgeour, C M, Smith, K, Stoward, P J, Rennie, M J, 1989, 'The effects of percutaneous electrical stimulation of atrophic human quadriceps on muscle composition, protein synthesis and contractile properties', *European Journal of Clinical Investigation* 19: 206–212

Gibson, J N A, Smith, K, Rennie, M J, 1988, 'Prevention of disuse muscle atrophy by means of electrical stimulation: maintenance of protein synthesis', *The Lancet* 2: 767–770

Gould, N, Donnermeyer, D, Gammon, G G, Pope, M, Ashikaga, T, 1983, 'Transcutaneous muscle stimulation to retard disuse atrophy after open meniscectomy', *Clinical Orthopaedics and Related Research* 178: 190–197

Hainaut, K, Duchateau, J, 1992, 'Neuromuscular electrical stimulation and voluntary exercise', *Sports Medicine* 14(2): 100–113

Halbach, J W, Straus, D, 1980, 'Comparison of electro-myo stimulation to isokinetic training in increasing power of the knee extensor mechanism', *Journal of Orthopaedic & Sports Physical Therapy* 2(1): 20–24

Johnson, D H, Thurston, P, Ashcroft, P J, 1977, 'The Russian technique of faradism in the treatment of chondromalacia patellae', *Physiotherapy Canada* 29(5): 266–268

Kramer, J F, 1987, 'Effect of electrical muscle stimulation current frequencies on isometric knee extension torque', *Physical Therapy* 67: 31–38

Lake, D A, 1992, 'Neuromuscular electrical stimulation: an overview and its application in the treatment of sports injuries', *Sports Medicine* 13(5): 320–336

Moreau, D, Dubots, P, Boggio, V, Guilland, J C, Cometti, G, 1995, 'Effects of electro-myostimulation and strength training on muscle soreness, muscle damage and sympathetic activation', *Journal of Sports Sciences* 13: 95–100

Morrissey, M C, Brewster, C E, Shields, C L, Brown, M, 1985, 'The effects of electrical stimulation of the quadriceps during postoperative knee immobilization', *American Journal of Sports Medicine* 13: 40–45

Nix, W A, Vrbová, G, 1986, *Electrical Stimulation and Neuromuscular Disorders*, Springer-Verlag, Heidelberg

Selkowitz, D M, 1985, 'Improvement in isometric strength of the quadriceps femoris muscle after training with electrical stimulation', *Physical Therapy* 65(2): 186–196

Sinacore, D R, 1990, 'Type II fiber activation with electrical stimulation: a preliminary report', *Physical Therapy* 70(7): 416–422

Sisk, T D, Stralka, S W, Deering, M B, et al., 1987, 'Effect of electrical stimulation on quadriceps strength after reconstructive surgery of the anterior cruciate ligament', *American Journal of Sports Medicine* 15: 215–219

Snyder-Mackler, L, Delitto, A, Stralka, S W, Bailey, S L, 1994, 'Use of electrical stimulation to enhance recovery of quadriceps femoris muscle force production in patients following anterior cruciate ligament reconstruction', *Physical Therapy* 74(10): 901–907

Thériault, R, Boulay, M R, Thériault, G, Simoneau, J-A, 1996, 'Electrical stimulation-induced changes in performance and fiber type proportion of human knee extensor muscles', *European Journal of Applied Physiology* 74: 311–317

Trimble, M H, Enoka, R M, 1991, 'Mechanisms underlying the training effects associated with neuromuscular electrical stimulation', *Physical Therapy* 71: 273–282

Wadey, V M, Knight, K, 1989, 'Four week training of quadriceps strength with electrical muscle stimulation and the isotonic DAPRE technique', *The Journal*, Canadian Athletic Trainers' Association, Spring/Summer: 14–20

Wigerstad-Lossing, I, Grimby, G, Jonsson, T, Morelli, B, Peterson, L, Renström, P, 1988, 'Effects of electrical muscle stimulation combined with voluntary contraction after knee ligament surgery', *Medicine and Science in Sports and Exercise* 20: 93–98

Williams, J G P, Street, M, 1976, 'Sequential faradism in quadriceps rehabilitation', *Physiotherapy* 62(8): 252–254

Rehabilitation and remedial exercises

Ainslie, T R, Beard, D J, 1996, 'Quantification of quadriceps passive resistance using isokinetic dynamometry', *Physiotherapy* 82(11): 628–630

Albert, M, 1991, *Eccentric Muscle Training in Sports and Orthopaedics*, Churchill Livingstone, Edinburgh

Alter, M J, 1996, *Science of Flexibility*, Human Kinetics, Champaign, Illinois, 2nd Edn

Antich, T J, Brewster, C E, 1986, 'Modification of quadriceps femoris muscle exercises during knee rehabilitation', *Physical Therapy* 66: 1246–1251

Appen, E L, Duncan, P W, 1986, 'Strength relationship of the knee musculature: effects of gravity and sport', *Journal of Orthopaedic & Sports Physical Therapy* 7: 232–235

Arvidsson, I, Eriksson, E, Haggmark, T, Johnson, R, 1981, 'Isokinetic thigh muscle strength after ligament reconstruction in the knee joint: results from a 5–10 year follow-up after reconstruction of the anterior cruciate ligament in the knee joint', *International Journal of Sports Medicine* 2: 7–11

Baechle, T R (ed.), 1994, *Essentials of Strength Training and Conditioning*, Human Kinetics, Champaign, Illinois

Basmajian, J V (ed.), 1984, *Therapeutic Exercise*, Williams and Wilkins, Baltimore, Maryland

Beard, D J, Zavatsky, A B, Murray, D W, Dowdall, M J, O'Connor, J J, 1994, 'Is leg-lifting in full extension safe following anterior cruciate ligament reconstruction?' *Physiotherapy* 80(7): 437–438

Brodowicz, G R, Welsh, R, Wallis, J, 1996, 'Comparison of stretching with ice, stretching with heat, or stretching alone on hamstring flexibility', *Journal of Athletic Training* 31(4): 324–327

Curl, W, Markey, K, Mitchell, W, 1983, 'Agility training following anterior cruciate ligament reconstruction', *Clinical Orthopaedics and Related Research* 172: 133–136

Dvir, Z, 1995, *Isokinetics. Muscle Testing, Interpretation, and Clinical Applications*, Churchill Livingstone International, New York, Edinburgh, London, Melbourne, Tokyo

Eriksson, E, 1981, 'Rehabilitation of muscle function after sports injury', *International Journal of Sports Medicine* 2: 1–6

Eriksson, E, 1996, 'The scientific basis of rehabilitation', *American Journal of Sports Medicine* 24(6) Suppl.: 525–527

Fisher, N M, Pendergast, D R, Gresham, G E, et al., 1991, 'Muscle rehabilitation: its effects on muscular and functional performance of patients with knee osteo-arthritis', *Archives of Physical Medicine and Rehabilitation* 72: 367–374

Grimby, G, Gustafsson, E, Peterson, L, Renström, P, 1980, 'Quadriceps function and training after knee ligament surgery', *Medicine and Science in Sport and Exercise* 12: 70–75

Hakkinen, K, 1989, 'Neuromuscular and hormonal adaptations during strength and power training', *Journal of Sports Medicine and Physical Fitness* 29: 9–26

Hall, L, Williams, J, 1989, 'The use of isokinetics in rehabilitation', *Physiotherapy* 75(10): 737–740

Hanten, W P, Schulthies, S S, 1990, 'Exercise effect on electromyographic activity of the vastus medialis oblique and vastus lateralis muscles', *Physical Therapy* 70: 9

Higgins, S, 1991, 'Motor control acquisition', *Physical Therapy* 71(2): 123–139

Ho, S S W, Illgen, R L, Meyer, R W, Torok, P J, Cooper, M D, Reider, B, 1995, 'Comparison of various icing times in decreasing bone metabolism and blood flow in the knee', *American Journal of Sports Medicine* 23(1): 74–76

Hurley, M V, Newham, D J, 1993, 'The influence of arthrogenous muscle inhibition on quadriceps rehabilitation of patients with early, uni-lateral osteo-arthritic knees', *British Journal of Rheumatology* 32: 127–131

Hutton, R S, Atwater, S W, 1992, 'Acute and chronic adaptations of muscle proprioceptors in response to increased use', *Sports Medicine* 14(6): 406–421

Ihara, H, Nakayama, A, 1986, 'Dynamic joint control training for knee ligament injuries', *American Journal of Sports Medicine* 14(4): 309–315

Ivy, J L, Withers, R T, Brose, G, Maxwell, B D, Costill, D L, 1981, 'Isokinetic

contractile properties of the quadriceps with relation to fiber types',
European Journal of Applied Physiology 47: 247–255

Kaufman, K R, An, K N, Litchy, W J, et al., 1991, 'Dynamic joint forces
during knee isokinetic exercise', *American Journal of Sports Medicine* 19:
305–316

Keskula, D R, 1996, 'Clinical implications of eccentric exercise in sports
medicine', *Journal of Sport Rehabilitation* 5(4): 321–329

Knight, K, 1995, *Cryotherapy in Sport Injury Management*, Human Kinetics,
Champaign, Illinois

Kreindler, H, Lewis, B B, Rush, S, et al., 1989, 'Effects of three exercise
protocols on strength of persons with osteo-arthritis of the knee', *Topics in
Geriatric Rehabilitation* 4: 32–39

LaChance, P, 1995, 'Plyometric exercise', *Strength and Conditioning* 17(4):
16–23

Lephart, S M, Pincivero, D M, Giraldo, J L, Fu, F H, 1997, 'The role of
proprioception in the management and rehabilitation of athletic injuries',
American Journal of Sports Medicine 25(1): 130–137

Li, R C T, Maffulli, N, Hsu, Y C, Chan, K M, 1996, 'Isokinetic strength of
the quadriceps and hamstrings and functional ability of anterior cruciate
ligament deficient knees in recreational athletes', *British Journal of Sports
Medicine* 30: 161–164

Lutz, G E, Palmitier, R A, An, K N, Chao, E Y S, 1991, 'Closed kinetic chain
exercises for athletes after reconstruction of the anterior cruciate ligament',
Medicine and Science in Sports and Exercise 24(4): 569

Lutz, G E, Palmitier, R A, An, K N, et al., 1993, 'Comparison of tibiofemoral
joint forces during open-kinetic-chain and closed-kinetic-chain exercises',
Journal of Bone and Joint Surgery 75A: 732–739

Marks, R, 1993, 'Quadriceps strength training for osteo-arthritis of the knee:
a literature review and analysis', *Physiotherapy* 79(1): 13–18

Marks, R, 1994, 'Quadriceps exercises for osteo-arthritis of the knee – a
single case study comparing short-term versus long-term training effects',
Physiotherapy 80(4): 195–199

Nyland, J, Brosky, T, Currier, D, Nitz, A, Caborn, D, 1994, 'Review of the
afferent neural system of the knee and its contribution to motor learning',
Journal of Orthopaedic and Sports Physical Therapy 19(1): 2–11

O'Sullivan, S B, 1994, *Physical Rehabilitation, Assessment and Treatment*,
F A Davis Co, Philadelphia

Palmitier, R A, Kainan, A, Scott, S G, Chao, E Y S, 1991, 'Kinetic chain
exercise in knee rehabilitation', *Sports Medicine* 11(6): 402–413

Perrin, D H, 1993, *Exercise and Assessment*, Human Kinetics Publishers,
Illinois

Pincivero, D M, Lephart, S M, Karunakara, R G, 1997, 'Effects of rest interval on isokinetic strength and functional performance after short term high intensity training', *British Journal of Sports Medicine* 31: 229–234

Pincivero, D M, Lephart, S M, Karunakara, R G, 1997, 'The relation between open and closed kinematic chain assessment of knee strength and functional performance', *Clinical Journal of Sports Medicine* 7: 11–16

Rice, M A, Bennett, J G, Ruhling, R O, 1995, 'Comparison of two exercises on VMO and VL EMG activity and force production', *Isokinetics and Exercise Science* 5: 61–67

Rothstein, J M, Lamb, R L, Mayhew, T P, 1987, 'Clinical uses of isokinetics', *Physical Therapy* 67(12): 1840–1844

Sale, D, 1988, 'Neural adaptations to resistance training', *Medicine and Science in Sports and Exercise* 20(5): 135–145

Sargeant, A J, Kernell, D (eds), 1993, *Neuromuscular Fatigue*, Amsterdam Faculty of Human Movement Sciences (ISBN 0 444 85763 X)

Stiene, H A, Brosky, T, Reinking, M F, Nyland, J, Mason, M B, 1996, 'A comparison of closed kinetic chain and isokinetic joint isolation exercise in patients with patellofemoral pain dysfunction', *Journal of Orthopaedic & Sports Physical Therapy* 24(3): 136–141

Stokes, M, Young, A, 1984, 'Investigations of quadriceps inhibition: implications for clinical practice', *Physiotherapy* 70(11): 425–428

Stokes, M, Young, A, 1984, 'The contribution of reflex inhibition to arthrogenous muscle weakness', *Clinical Science* 67: 7–14

Tegner, Y, 1990, 'Strength training in the rehabilitation of cruciate ligament tears', *Sports Medicine* 9(2): 129–136

Threlkeld, A, Horn, T, Wojtowicz, G, Rooney, J, Shapiro, R, 1989, 'Kinematics, ground reaction force and muscle balance produced by backward running', *Journal of Orthopaedic & Sports Physical Therapy* 11(2): 56–63

Timm, K, 1987, 'Investigation of the physiological overflow effect from speed-specific isokinetic activity', *Journal of Orthopaedic & Sports Physical Therapy* 9(3): 106–110

Tippett, S R, Voight, M L, 1995, *Functional Progressions for Sport Rehabilitation*, Human Kinetics, Champaign, Illinois

Wawrzyniak, J R, Tracy, J E, Catizone, P V, Storrow, R R, 1996, 'Effect of closed chain exercise on quadriceps femoris peak torque and functional performance', *Journal of Athletic Training* 31(4): 335–340

Wilk, K E, Escamilla, R F, Fleisig, G S, Barrentine, S W, Andrews, J R, Boyd, M L, 1996, 'A comparison of tibiofemoral joint forces and electromyographic activity during open and closed kinetic chain exercises', *American Journal of Sports Medicine* 24(4): 518–527

Wilk, K E, Simoneau, G, McGraw, J, 1993, 'The electromyographic activity of the quadriceps femoris vastus medialis/lateralis ratio during squats, leg press, and knee extension exercises', *Physical Therapy* 73: 580

Wyse, J P, Mercer, T H, Gleeson, N P, 1994, 'Time-of-day dependence of isokinetic leg strength and associated interday variability', *British Journal of Sports Medicine* 28(3): 167–170

Index

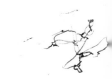